SECRETS OF SASSY, SAVVY SENIORS

AGING LIKE
ROYALTY ROADMAP

SECRETS OF SASSY, SAVVY SENIORS

DR. NAKEISHA RAQUEL RODGERS

publish
your gift

DEDICATION

To my precious parents, Hermon and Sylvia, who through their tireless sacrifices loved me and supported my every endeavor. Your wisdom gave me the foundation to cultivate all the gifts God placed inside me.

To my darling sister, Kathrina Rodgers Munroe. You always spoke greatness over my life. Your unconditional love for our parents inspires me every day.

TABLE OF CONTENTS

Introduction 1

PART 1: THE ROADMAP TO AGING LIKE
ROYALTY 5

Chapter 1: Preparing for the Royal Years:
Understanding Normal Aging 7

Chapter 2: How Savvy Seniors Select Their
Physician 41

Chapter 3: Why Savvy Seniors Need a Geriatrician 49

Chapter 4: Assembling the Royal Court: Key
Partnerships as You Age 61

Chapter 5: Leaving a Lasting Honorable Legacy 69

PART 2: THE ROYAL SECRETS OF
LONGEVITY 73

Chapter 6: Geriatrician/Patient Relationship 75

Chapter 7: There's No Place Like Home: Preventing
Hospitalizations 79

Chapter 8: Unlocking the Royal Codes: Savvy
Seniors Know Their Numbers 89

Chapter 9: Navigating the Hospital System 97

Chapter 10: How My Sassy Seniors Taught Me
to Age Like Royalty 107

Conclusion 121

Afterword 123

References.. 125

About the Author 127

INTRODUCTION

I grew up on the beautiful archipelagic islands of the Bahamas. Given the moniker "the place where God lives," by the late great Dr. Myles Munroe, the Bahamas is a majestic gem nestled merely fifty miles off the coast of Florida. With a population of nearly 400,000, it has produced some of the most talented figures to grace the world stage.

My parents enrolled me in Our Lady's Catholic Primary school. Faith was important. There, we routinely attended Friday morning Mass. Albeit mandatory, this consistent exposure would become paramount to my own personal walk with God and would later influence my work ethic.

As a student, I only remembered wanting to be of service. As my mother recalls, I also had a powerful connection—seniors. At age six, I would scrummage for all the change I could find to go to the bakery after school. After twenty long painstaking minutes, my parents usually discovered that I was deeply engrossed in a conversation with the bakery's proprietor, Mr. B.

I can still envision him. His smooth dark skin highlighted his white, majestically coiled crown of grey curls. Dark aging spots were intricately arranged on his face. They flawlessly framed his big hazel eyes and huge warm smile. "And how was your day today, little lady?" At the tender age of six, I would recite all the exciting big words I was taught by my second-grade teacher, Mrs. Barbara Moseley-Gray. I remembered feeling so valued that he, approaching his seventies, would take the time to listen to the second-grade adventures of a six-year-old. He stood as a pillar of wisdom, and I latched onto his every word.

Fast forward to the year 2000. I had decided to pursue a Bachelor of Science in Biology at Acadia University in Nova Scotia, Canada. One day, a normal stroll to Wolfville Elms started me on an amazing trajectory. I felt an electric surge of excitement when I started volunteering as a helper at this skilled nursing facility.

I volunteered with the arts and crafts department, cleaned tables, hand-fed residents, and visited with them. A ninety-year-old resident recounted how she learnt a close family relative had perished in the Titanic. I was destined to find my purpose and gifting in the field of geriatrics. It is not just a medical subspecialty; it is literally and figuratively my life.

On November 30, 2020, I received the phone call that would change my life. "Keisha, I didn't want to tell you, but your daddy has not been feeling well and wants to see the doctor!" Reliving that day, I remember the nervous undertones in her voice.

My heart immediately sank into my chest, and it skipped several beats. Large pellets of sweat engulfed my palms so quickly that the cell phone began to slip from my clutch. I sat paralyzed with fear in my study while my mind began to teem with uncertainty. My eyes later welled up with salty tears that started to stream down my cheeks.

Over the next few days, I asked God to arm me with the courage and strength to face whatever this was. Besides my faith, the only person with whom I could be vulnerable was my big sister Kathrina. She was alone in the Bahamas while I was thousands of miles away. Nevertheless, we worked as a cohesive duo *7681*, a symbolism of our birth years, to ensure that my father got all the necessary testing and procedures. By the grace of God, our father was all right. Though I was in the medical field and my sister was an exceptional caregiver, there were still a few issues we had to address, albeit the team administering his care did their best.

From this experience, I was convinced that my life's purpose was helping other seniors and their caregivers get the medical tools they need to age with poise and dignity. My sister and I are not just health aficionados but are simply two doting daughters who absolutely adore, honor, and cherish our parents.

We have been there and thankfully by God's grace we have each other. Our mission is to equip devoted caregivers with spiritual and educational tools so they too can help their loved ones age like royalty.

When I reminisce on why I pursued geriatrics, I fondly remember graduation night at my internal medicine residency program in Bridgeport, Connecticut. My mentor, Dr. Yaw Adjepong, and critical care attending, Dr. John Paul Ayala, whom I both deeply respect and admire, looked me stark in the eyes and told me, "Nakeisha, there's nobody else more suited to become the Geriatric Maven. You go out there and do it!" And so, with faith and resilience, I am committed to mapping out the journey to successful aging. I am excited for you to join me!

PART 1:

THE ROADMAP
TO AGING
LIKE ROYALTY

—◦—

CHAPTER 1

PREPARING FOR THE ROYAL YEARS: UNDERSTANDING NORMAL AGING

There are numerous theories on aging. As the body chronically ages, all organ systems are affected. Many seniors are told to helplessly embrace their ailments as a part of the normal aging process. "Well, you do know that you are elderly, just be thankful that you are alive." This sentiment has caused many a well-intentioned relative to ascribe normal aging to actual disease states that are not a part of aging. So, before you can age like the true boss that you are, you must know the answer to this time-honored question, "Is this symptom normal for my age?" In this chapter, get out your pen and paper and take notes on what constitutes normal aging in each system of the body.

MEDICATIONS AND AGING

As we age, the number of neuron or brain cells decreases. The process of encoding, storing, and retrieving memories is affected. It is common for patients to start asking those time-honored questions: "Hey, where'd I put my keys?" or "What's your name again?" Muscle mass goes down while adipose fat tissues increase. This not only affects the sexy senior who fondly reminisces on the good ol' days when he could display his rippling six pack abs, but it also leads to various effects of medications on the body.

Since the aging body has a greater percentage of fat or adipose tissue, physicians who care for savvy seniors must be extremely meticulous about the way they prescribe medications. In much the same way that a treasured recipe is dear to the heart of a sous chef, the Beers Criteria for Potentially Inappropriate Medication Use in Older Adults (commonly called the Beers list) is paramount to the practice of the geriatrician (Durso, et al. 2013).

This list was pioneered in 1991 by the late great geriatric extraordinaire Dr. Mark Beers. It has since been revised posthumously by his successors. The list was most recently revised in 2019 and outlines potentially inappropriate medications in the elderly. It is broadly divided into four categories. The first reviews medications that can adversely affect various organ systems. The second outlines medications that can exacerbate certain syndromes or diseases. The third classification outlines medications that must be used cautiously. The fourth highlights certain medications that should not be prescribed together.

Let me be clear. There are some cases where a medication on the Beers list is needed. The list does not explicitly ban the use of medications on it. It is an important reminder for geriatricians to pause and review their reasons for prescribing a medication. Savvy seniors enjoy thoughtful, enriching discussions about the Beers list and want to minimize potentially appropriate medications.

Drugs can be broadly divided into two categories— lipophilic or fat soluble and hydrophilic water soluble. In layman's terms, some medications are fat loving and dissolve easier in fatty environments while other medications are better absorbed in tissues that are predominantly fluid.

Lipophilic medications include certain benzodiazepines such as valium. These medications have a longer period of duration in the body with a prolonged effect. Benzodiazepines do have their place in providing anxiolytic relief in the short term, however, as time goes on, escalating doses are often required to get the same effect. This can lead to habit-forming dependencies.

The effects of this particular class of medications can be more profound and pronounced as a person ages. From a pathophysiologic perspective, seniors are more likely to experience the untoward effects. These include greater sedation leading to a heightened risk of respiratory depression, falls, and fractures. Physicians who are knowledgeable about these intricate changes in aging recognize this and always educate their patients about it. Once properly educated, savvy seniors can make an informed decision about their medication regimen and possible adverse effects.

CARDIOVASCULAR SYSTEM AND AGING

Heart disease is the leading cause of death in male and female patients over sixty-five. As the body ages, the contractility of the blood vessels and the heart muscle is reduced. This process is typically the result of hypertension. The US Preventative Disease Task Force defines hypertension in seniors as a systolic value over 150 and diastolic value over 90. The 8th Joint National Committee, which evaluates hypertension, also considers hypertension to be any value greater than 150/90 in a senior over sixty-five (Durso et al. 2013).

Ever wondered why hypertension has the notorious moniker, the silent killer? Persons who live with years and years of untreated blood pressure set themselves up for structural changes in the chambers or ventricles of the heart. The muscle thickens in a process called hypertrophy. You're probably asking, "Well, what's so bad with a thickened heart muscle, shouldn't it help my heart to pump more successfully?" Well, after months and years of hypertrophy, a person can develop abnormal arrythmias such as atrial fibrillation. They can also develop diastolic dysfunction.

In layman's terms, with diastolic dysfunction, the heart muscle becomes so thick that filling of the coronary blood vessels during diastole is compromised. The coronaries are the blood vessels that feed and nourish the heart muscle. When the heart muscle is starved of important nutrients, patients develop angina or chest pain. Additionally, blood backs up in the heart, analogous to a traffic jam. Blood must seek another recourse. So where does it go? You've guessed it! Blood is diverted backwards from the left side of the heart into the lungs. Blood pools in the lungs resulting in noticeable shortness of breath with exertion. If this continues unabated, the person becomes short of breath even at rest!

If the "traffic jam" becomes greater, the patient will develop failure in the right side of the heart. He or she will notice swelling in the lower extremities, abdomen, and even distended neck veins. Patients who present with these findings are eventually diagnosed with congestive heart failure.

Congestive heart disease is a leading cause of recurrent hospitalizations in seniors. Throughout my practice, I can't tell you how many patients and families are battling this disease without the secrets they need for combat. Many patients are advised that persons with congestive heart failure must avoid a salty diet, but only savvy seniors really understand what a low sodium diet means.

A low salt diet typically has 2000 mg. sodium or less. That sounds like a lot. Savvy seniors understand that 2000 mg. is not as large as it seems. One teaspoon contains close to 2000 mg. of sodium. Savvy seniors are knowledgeable about how to read labels when they trek to the grocery store. They creatively replace their saltshakers with mouthwatering herbs and spices and transition to seasonings sans sodium like Mrs. Dash. They have met with their primary care physician, cardiologist, and dietitian to tweak their favorite soul food and traditional ethnic dishes, so they do not have to sacrifice a trip to the hospital for good ol' flavor.

Beyond their blood pressure and diuretic pills, the one prized possession of all savvy seniors with congestive heart disease is a scale. All seniors know their dry weight by heart, no pun intended. This dry weight is their ideal body weight when they are completely symptom free. Savvy seniors weigh themselves faithfully every morning after emptying their bladders and before consuming a meal. If their weight increases in twenty-four hours, two to three pounds above their dry weight, they can immediately increase their diuretic pill, oftentimes, Lasix, to remove this extra fluid. This prevents an exacerbation of congestive cardiac disease and an emergency room visit or hospitalization.

If the eyes are the window to the soul, the heart is the storehouse of the emotions. Cardiology is an ever-evolving specialty with breaking developments every day. Approximately 10 percent of all seniors over seventy-five have an arrythmia called *atrial fibrillation*. Why am I telling you about atrial fibrillation? Failure to diagnose and properly manage it can have drastic and even deadly consequences. Medications to prevent complications from atrial fibrillation are advertised repeatedly on television. You've probably been bombarded by quite a few anticoagulant brand names including Eliquis and Xarelto. These medications are used to prevent a fatal stroke.

Atrial fibrillation is an irregular heartbeat in which the smaller atrial chambers beat out of synchrony with the larger ventricles. In simple terms the atria begin to "quiver" rather that contract. Irregularly conducted beats eventually escape down the pathway to the larger ventricle chambers. The heartbeat is out of sync leading to palpitations, shortness of breath, and dizziness. I perform electrocardiograms regularly on all my seniors especially those reporting vague symptoms of unexplainable fatigue as this may be the only clue to a diagnosis of atrial fibrillation. If there is cause for concern, I will follow up with an echocardiogram. This is a painless, noninvasive ultrasound of the heart performed by a technician and interpreted by a cardiologist. The echocardiogram provides important information about the anatomy and contractility of the heart.

One of the most feared complications of atrial fibrillation is a cardioembolic stroke. Strokes from atrial fibrillation are more devastating than those which result from years of high cholesterol. When the atrial chambers fibrillate and quiver, blood has time to pool and form clots that eventually enter the ventricle. When the ventricle contracts, the blood clots are fired in a flurry of showers through the aorta which eventually connects to the arteries in the neck. One important vessel in the neck is the internal carotid artery which eventually connects to the posterior retina via the ophthalmic artery.

Patients experience temporary visual loss or the sensation of a curtain falling in their visual field a condition termed *amaurosis fugax*. If a clot travels from the internal carotid to the middle cerebral artery the person, can develop unilateral weakness and even dysarthria if the clot obstructs blood flow in the left middle cerebral artery. Many patients prefer to suffer a heart attack or acute myocardial infarction over a stroke cerebrovascular accident. Why? Independence is one of the greatest treasures of the sassy and savvy senior. He or she often dreads the loss of mobility and functionality that a devastating stroke can bring.

Decades of poor eating habits can eventually take their toll on a senior. Strokes termed cerebrovascular accidents are one of the most feared consequences of high cholesterol and hypertension. The good old adage, "an apple a day keeps the doctor away," continues to ring true. Many patients recognize the relationship of high cholesterol to a stroke, but some may feel powerless to improve their numbers simply because of a lack of knowledge.

I order a fasting test on my patients called a lipid panel. This test calculates my patient's total cholesterol, which should ideally be under 250. The test then surmises the patient's triglyceride level. This is largely affected by diet. Food and animal products high in trans fats can lead to a very high triglyceride value which can spell disaster for a patient's blood vessels.

Another component of the lipid panel is the LDL. The LDL, or low-density lipoprotein, contributes to blockages throughout the body's arterial system. The HDL, or high-density lipoprotein, is beneficial. It helps to unclog the arteries by shuttling fat from the lining of the blood vessels back to the liver for breakdown. So, are you saying that not all cholesterol is bad? I am saying a resounding yes! All cholesterol is not created equal.

The goal of healthy eating is to reduce the consumption of processed and animal-based products which can increase the triglycerides and LDL levels. My savvy seniors understand that they need to keep their HDL high and their LDL low as possible under 70. HDL levels can be increased by consuming vegetables and nuts and by exercising. Patient should be encouraged to participate in thirty minutes of physical activity at least five days per week. Quarantining during COVID-19 has sparked my patients' ingenuity and creativity. Some have substituted their grocery store can goods for weights, their bath towels for stretch cords, and the steps in their living room for an elliptical. Necessity has truly been the mother of invention!

Of note, as a geriatrician I would be remiss if I didn't share one important detail. While we strive to ensure that the total cholesterol is kept low, too much of a good thing can also have consequences. Geriatricians get alarmed if their patient's total cholesterol is under 160. This diagnosis is termed hypocholesteremia. In the context of unintentional weight loss of greater than ten pounds in six months, reduced gait speed, and fatigue, hypocholesteremia may signal the alarm for undernutrition and a potential underlying malignancy. This is one of the reasons savvy seniors must involve their physicians in the interpretation and discussion of all phlebotomy results.

RESPIRATORY SYSTEM AND AGING

Many of you may remember and love the iconic '80s Berlin classic *Take My Breath Away*. It was the unforgettable soundtrack for the Tom Cruise movie *Top Gun*. When it comes to aging, Berlin's anthem does ring true. The amount of air or tidal volume we inhale each second decreases with aging. Lung tissue also becomes less compliant. The cartilage supporting the ribs become stiffer. On the surface this change may seem innocuous, but it can explain why breathing becomes even more challenging for older patients with superimposed lung illnesses such as asthma, chronic bronchitis, or emphysema. It is the reason why persons over sixty-five are at greater risk for COVID-19 pulmonary complications.

The lung is aerated by millions of grapelike sacs called alveoli. Fewer and fewer of these sacs fill as we age. This leads to flattening or atelectasis. I often explain this to my patients as having more deflated air balloons. These deflated air balloons can become a reservoir for infection, especially in patients with a propensity for developing aspiration pneumonias.

Outside of infections like bacterial pneumonia and COVID-19, there remains one key activity that increases the risk of lung disease. What is it? Well, I'm glad you asked. Tobacco use remains a leading cause of chronic lung conditions. "Well, Dr. Rodgers, I don't smoke but my husband does in the next room." Most patients appreciate the damage of tobacco use but some often do not recognize that second-hand smoke is just as deleterious.

When patients inhale, while they get the pleasurable effects of nicotine, they also get cancer-causing chemicals and tobacco. The free radicals in cigarette smoke inflame the airways. The airways try to protect themselves by secreting copious amounts of thick purulent mucus. This leads to a component of COPD (chronic obstructive pulmonary disease) termed chronic bronchitis. Many patients experience a chronic productive cough and wheezing. Think of living with severe chronic bronchitis each day as taking a deep breath through a tiny straw.

Tobacco use can set the stage for another variant of COPD termed emphysema. The free radicals in tobacco smoke damage the elastic connections between the grapelike alveolar sacs. The sacs are destroyed. The surface area available for the lungs to obtain oxygen is diminished. Patients get very winded with minimal activity. A stroll through the grocery store can seem like running a marathon. Eventually, patients may get so deconditioned and short of breath with end stage COPD that they must depend on an oxygen tank twenty-four hours daily.

It is estimated that approximately fifteen million people in the United States carry a diagnosis of COPD. About 10 percent of this population includes seniors over sixty-five. COPD is also responsible for roughly 20 percent of all hospitalizations in persons between sixty-five and seventy-five years of age. COPD exacerbations that result in ICU mechanical ventilation are associated with mortality rates between 11-46 percent (Durso et al. 2013). In this COVID-19 pandemic era, the significance of COPD in seniors cannot be downplayed. All patients with COPD are especially encouraged to practice social distancing, hand hygiene, and mask use. They are also urged to ensure that they are up to date on appropriate vaccines.

Lung health can be improved by daily aerobic exercise that helps to strengthen the pulmonary muscles. Patients can have their doctors order incentive spirometers. These are plastic, demarcated hand-held devices with a floating ball. The device has a mouthpiece through which the patient deeply inhales. The patient tries to elevate the floating ball with each breath. The markings correspond to the volume of air inhaled.

If you are savvy senior with a diagnosis of COPD, please talk to your doctor about enrolling in programs such as pulmonary rehabilitation. These programs are done in conjunction with physical and respiratory therapists to promote exercise and teach more effective breathing strategies. Savvy seniors with COPD are often familiar with the parameters of their pulmonary function testing and have this done annually to monitor the lung's ability. Ultimately, they recognize that they can reap the benefits of smoking cessation at any age. They also understand that lung function can be preserved by avoiding bronchial irritants in cigarettes, e-cigarettes, and vaping.

SENSORY SYSTEM AND AGING

As I continue to advance in my career, I remain mesmerized by the intricacy of the human body. Each organ system undergoes changes. The sensory system, including vision, hearing, taste, and smell, are all impacted by aging. The number of receptors responsible for each system declines.

Presbycusis is the medical term for age-related hearing loss. When the sensorineural nerve is affected, patients lose the ability to hear high pitched sounds. Many will have to dial up the volume on their television sets and on their cell phones. Many patients with hearing loss find it challenging to engage in conversations with background noises like crowded restaurants. They rely extensively on lip-reading.

It is important to have your ear canal inspected at each doctor appointment. Hearing loss may simply be the result of impaction by cerumen, or in layman's terms, earwax. A quick and painless syringe procedure in the office can restore a patient's hearing just like new! If the otoscope examination does not reveal impaction with cerumen, then the patient can be referred for an audiology examination. During this exam, he or she must distinguish the amplitude and frequency of various tones. This helps to determine if the sensorineural nerve is damaged in either ear. If sensorineural hearing loss is confirmed by an audiologist, the patient is prescribed appropriate hearing aids. The type and quality of hearing aids has completely advanced over the last few decades. Many insurances do not cover hearing aids, and these must be purchased out of pocket by the patient.

Taste and smell have risen to the forefront with the stark surge in COVID-19 cases. The virus is known to impair both sensory modalities in its victims. Taste and smell are critical in tickling and capturing a sassy senior's palate. As we age, we lose many taste receptors. Foods can become bland. Well-intentioned family members can become distraught as they struggle to satisfy the selective demands of their sassy seniors. "Mom only takes a small bite of her food and then she's done, she's going to lose weight, so what can we do?"

Once family members and patients are educated about the reduction in taste and olfactory receptors that occurs with normal aging, they can devise simple solutions to whetting their relative's appetite. Sweet taste receptors are the last to go. If there is no overt medical reason to restrict a patient's diet, I encourage patients to liberalize their diet. This allows for the addition of sweetened smoothies, along with nutritive supplements in between meals. In short, patients can relish savory highly flavored cuisines.

One important Bible verse that I really love from the New King James Bible is Hosea 4:6 "My people perish for lack of knowledge!" In the field of Geriatrics, we can take this verse quite literally. Loss of vision can wreak major havoc on a patient's ability and confidence in ambulating. Patients who develop challenges with their vision may start to develop the fear of falls leading them to restrict their mobility. This can further impact their mental and social wellbeing leading to feelings of isolation and depression.

All savvy seniors should be reminded to have an annual ophthalmologic examination. Annual examinations can help with early detection of many life-changing ocular diagnoses such as cataract formation, age related macular degeneration, and glaucoma.

LOVING THE SKIN YOU'RE IN AT EVERY AGE

The largest organ of the human body is also affected. "Which organ is that?" you may be asking. You guessed it! It is the skin. We have all heard the phrase, beauty is only skin deep. We live in a world where the Ponce de León quest for the fountain of youth will never stop. I am often intrigued by the dozens of infomercials which promise that their injection and cremes will deliver age-defying results. Some have incorporated home remedies, such as lemon juice and honey peels, to detoxify their skin.

The skin is the body's greatest barrier to damaging agents like the ultraviolet rays, micro-organisms, and trauma. The numbers of keratinocytes and melanocytes that add the lustrous hues to our hair also declines. This leads to graying. Attempts to combat it have driven the success of billion-dollar cosmetic empires like Loreal, Dark and Lovely, and Revlon, just to name a few.

The outermost level, called the epidermis, flattens as we age. The underlying supportive dermis atrophies, resulting in wrinkles and loss of tone, particularly in the arm regions. Dermatologists can augment the soft tissues of the face via injectable fillers. They try to remove wrinkles from the face by using neurotoxins like Botox, which relax the contracted muscles around the eyes that create crow's feet and wrinkles. Years of unfiltered exposure to harmful UV sunlight can lead to skin with a dry, leathery texture. Photodamage can also promote aging spots called lentigines. These spots are relatively benign and can be tan or dark in appearance. They are most commonly found on the face.

In addition to encouraging a yearly skin examination with a dermatologist, sexy, savvy, and sassy seniors are all educated about ways they can protect themselves from the scorching UV rays. They are taught about the benefits of wearing wide-brimmed hats and clothing, protective eye-wear, and using sunscreens that offer ultraviolet A and B protection. I stress this to my melanated patients of color to correct the misperception that pigmented skin does not require SPF support. All skin needs an extra ounce of tender, loving, SPF care!

THE AGING BLADDER

One of the questions that I get a lot from patients and their families is, "why do I have to urinate so much as I get older?" The frequent, involuntary passage of urine is termed incontinence. It is not entirely the result of normal aging. Only 5-15 percent of community-dwelling seniors are truly incontinent. As we age, the storage capacity of the bladder is reduced. The bladder opens into the urethra. In females, the urethra is a miniature orifice antecedent to the vagina. Urethral closure is reinforced by a sling-like mesh of pelvic floor muscles. These pelvic floor muscles weaken with obesity and multiple births. This makes it harder for the urethra to close, increasing the risk of incontinence in females.

The male urethra is housed in the penis. It originates from the base of bladder and travels through the prostate. Men with enlarged or hypertrophied prostates can develop difficulty with the flow of urine called dribbling. Conversely, prostate enlargement may also cause irritative symptoms leading to urinary frequency. In both sexes, aging is associated with reduced bladder storage.

Urinary incontinence can stem from several conditions. It can be increased by certain medications like diuretics. It can result from ingestion of bladder stimulants, like caffeine, close to bedtime.

The best approach to treating urinary incontinence is examining the patient's lifestyle habits. I encourage my patients to keep a diary of their fluid intake and fluid output for at least seven days. The patient records the amount and type of fluid consumed and the time of day. Hindsight is usually 20/20. A eureka lightbulb normally goes off as patients start to realize that they are sipping from a glass of water on the bedside dresser throughout the night. "Well doc, it's just that my mouth gets so dry from my pills, that's why I keep some water near my bedstand." This reasoning is understandable but does have the adverse effect of multiple bedtime and early morning treks to the bathroom.

In such cases, geriatricians like myself immediately find alternatives for medications known to have anticholinergic or drying properties. Additionally, I have my patients trade their bedtime glass of water for oral lubricants such as Biotene spray and Biotene mouthwashes. I cannot tell you how great of an improvement they get from these simple tweaks.

From their fluid diary, some patients also may realize that they are ingesting particularly larger quantities of caffeinated beverages like sodas, teas, and coffee than they had estimated. Once they see the evidence in black and white, many will appreciate the profound effect that excess caffeine has on urinary frequency. I particularly enjoy using the fluid diary because it fosters a sense of partnership between my patients and I. Anecdotally, patients who are more engaged in their care are generally more committed to executing their care plan.

Geriatricians classify urinary incontinence into several causes. The most common is urge incontinence, which has become popularized by the catchy "gotta go, gotta go" television jingle. This type of incontinence stems from overactivity of the detrusor bladder muscle. If behavioral techniques are minimally successful, patients are prescribed drugs from either of two major classes of medications. The first group, called antimuscarinics, include tradenames like Detrol. These medications block the overactive detrusor muscle receptors. The biggest side effects are constipation or reduced oral secretions. Persons generally report dry mouth that is alleviated by mouth washes and sprays like Biotene. The second class of incontinence medications relaxes the detrusor muscle using a different pharmacologic pathway. The prototype is called Myrbetriq. It must be used with caution in patients with baseline hypertension.

The next most common type of incontinence is stress, as its name suggests. Female patients report involuntary passage of urine with stressors that increase intra-abdominal pressure, such as coughing or laughing. This form of incontinence stems from deconditioning of the supportive pelvic floor muscles. It is best treated with the use of Kegel exercises. Females repeatedly contract their pelvic muscles. This can be down covertly throughout the day. Some patients have a mixed presentation with features of both urge and stress incontinence.

Another important type of incontinence is overflow incontinence. This occurs when urine begins to leak from an already distended bladder. Overflow incontinence demands a judicious search for all potential culprits. The most feared is damage to the parasympathetic nerves that innervate the bladder. Damage to the nerves may stem from trauma, malignancy, neurodegenerative lesions, or autonomic conditions like poorly controlled diabetes mellitus. Patients with overflow incontinence generally have over 200ml of residual urine volume left in the bladder even after they have voided. These patients sometimes require intermittent or chronic foley catheterizations.

The last type of incontinence is functional. Sassy seniors who are fiercely independent and mobile will rarely experience this. Functional incontinence is most pronounced in hospitalized seniors or those residing in chronic care facilities who have lost their degree of ambulation. Such patients respond to prompted voiding where they are invited to go the restroom every two hours.

Whatever the etiology, urinary incontinence wreaks the same consequences on affected seniors. Many respond by altering their day-to-day consumption of fluids. Others have cleverly utilized undergarment pads to prevent soiling. Incontinence can reduce a senior's sense of independence. They may decline opportunities to attend socials for fear of lacking timely access to a restroom. They may become emotionally and mentally distressed by the fact that their caregivers must launder their undergarments and linens much more frequently. Urinary incontinence has been cited as a major cause for long term care placement.

Studies suggest that less than 50 percent of seniors will inform their doctors of concerns about urinary incontinence because they feel it comes with the territory of normal aging (Durso et al. 2013). Geriatricians of sassy, savvy, and sexy seniors understand this innocent misconception. They make it a priority to ask about urinary incontinence at least annually during their geriatric assessment.

SLEEP CYCLE AND AGING

I would be remiss if I didn't talk about the changes in sleep that occur with normal aging. Sleep hygiene is a common concern among savvy seniors and their caregivers. "Mom just does not sleep at night and then she's knocked out during the day!" As we lay our heads down to drift off into our dreams of fantasy, our body enters several stages. These are divided into rapid eye movement (REM) and non-REM. REM sleep is the stage where we are transported into our utopian worlds and begin to dream. It also the deepest level of sleep where are bodies get the most rest and from which we feel most refreshed.

Research has shown that as we age, we experience lesser amounts of REM sleep. Seniors feel less rejuvenated when they awake. The stages of sleep become shorter. Many family members are amazed that their savvy senior can survive on so little amount of rest. If not engaged in purposeful activity, seniors may find that they nap more frequently throughout the day.

Insomnia is by far one of the most challenging, yet common, complaints. It is often impacted by so many underlying risk factors—lifestyle habits, incontinence, medication, and mood disorders, just to name a few. Insomnia can become so distressing and debilitating that some physicians may eventually resort to using more potent and sedating agents like benzodiazepines to treat insomnia. Again, let's be clear. No two physicians are the same.

Given the risk of geriatric syndromes, like falls that increase as we age, along with the decline in kidney and liver drug metabolism, I tend to err on the side of less sedating agents when treating patients with poor sleep hygiene.

Like the urinary incontinence, the diagnosis and management of insomnia requires some investigative detective work. I start with having patients describe a typical day. We discuss their activity, their liquid intake, even down to their favorite television shows. We explore their medical history to determine if there are any risks such as evening diuretics, evening caffeine, or stimulating medications such as Ritalin which are best taken by the early afternoon. With the pressures of COVID-19 and the accompanying isolation, insomnia can signal underlying depression. For this reason, I perform the GDS or Geriatric Depression Scale. It is comprised of fifteen questions that focus on a patient's sense of purpose. It is more sensitive for depression in seniors than the typical Patient Health Questionnaire-9 (PHQ-9). The latter asks about more subjective symptoms, like appetite and concentration, which can be the result of underlying chronic disease.

COGNITION AND AGING

The most common disease that most of my patients are concerned about is dementia. It remains a hot topic, but there remains a big discrepancy in the understanding of what dementia really is. "Well, Mrs. X doesn't have dementia, she has Alzheimer's!"

When physicians use the term dementia, they are referring to the broad spectrum of disorders that affect at least two domains of a person's mental ability or cognition. The major domains of mental ability include the domains of memory, language, executive planning, visuospatial and abstract thinking. The deficit in two domains must affect the patient's ability to function independently.

As we get older, it is reasonable to forget where we place our keys or to forget a person's name. This is called normal aging. Along this spectrum emerges a state called mild cognitive impairment where the patient recognizes some challenges in memory, but they are still independent.

In comparison to mild cognitive impairment, patients with dementia have memory defects that complicate their ability to perform IADLS and ADLs. Doctors define IADLs as instrumental activities of daily living. IADLs include driving, cooking, laundry, paying bills in a timely manner, and organizing medications. When your doctor uses the term ADLs, he or she is enquiring about your ability to do more inherently simpler activities of daily living like bathing, grooming, and eating. Like our counterparts in other specialties, we geriatricians are also creatures of habit. We classify the stages of Alzheimer's dementia using the Reisberg Functional Assessment Staging Tool (FAST).

This tool has seven classifications. FAST 1 is a person with no functional impairment. FAST 2 is a patient with symptoms of normal aging. FAST 3 is a person with mild cognitive impairment. This person will have objective evidence of deficits in at least one or more domains. Patients at the level of FAST 4 develop some difficulty at work and at this point the term dementia is used. FAST 5 and 6 result in difficulties with grooming, bathing, and other ADLs. FAST 7 is the terminal phase of dementia. This is perhaps the toughest stage in the long goodbye. During this time, doctors and families tend to elicit the expertise of Hospice Specialists to support the patient and family. FAST 7 is further subdivided into six stages where a patient goes from speaking a few words to losing their ability to eat and interact meaningfully with verbal language.

A great number of persons can remain at the FAST 3 stage of mild cognitive impairment. So many times, I have encountered mild cognitive impairment (MCI) patients who are extremely concerned that they in fact have true dementia. While I try to assuage their fears that they are still performing their IADLs, and ADLs I emphasize the importance of charting their memory over time with brief in office memory tests like the MOCA.

This test called the Montreal Cognitive Assessment test was developed by McGill researcher Dr. Nasreddine. It analyzes the domains of language, executive function, attention, memory, and visuospatial function. It is scored out of thirty with twenty-six being a normal result. It has been translated into more than thirty-five languages globally. It has been adapted for visually impaired patients. It cannot be used alone to formally diagnose dementia but must be combined with collateral history from trusted caregivers along with the results of laboratory and brain imaging.

The MOCA test typically takes about ten minutes to administer. Interpreters of the results must be clinically certified because the results can have far reaching legal implications on a person's ability to remain employed and to drive.

The MOCA test is most useful in detecting mild cognitive impairment in patients who are highly intellectually functioning. It's a common arsenal in the geriatrician's diagnostic tool for mild cognitive screening. Approximately 12-15 percent of patients with MCI can progress to dementia over the course of three to five years. Geriatricians will perform the MOCA annually to chart our patient's performances. The results can provide further insight into the patient's strengths and areas for improvement.

There are several classes of dementia, and Alzheimer's is the most widely known. This particular dementia is most common in seniors after age sixty-five but can occur in those much younger. Patients that are diagnosed with early onset dementia may be sent for genetic testing for defects in proteins such as presenilin and apolipoprotein E (APOE).

To form a memory, the human brain must encode, store, and retrieve. This dynamic process primarily involves numerous intricate neuron cells and circuits that converge in the region of the brain termed the hippocampus. The cells in this region communicate with each other with the assistance of two important proteins. The first, called the *tau protein*, forms the backbone and structural support of the nerve cell. The second protein, *amyloid precursor protein*, is beautifully nestled in the communicating space or *synapse* between two cells.

Alzheimer's patients develop a defect in their tau protein. The structural integrity of the neuron or nerve cell is compromised. The cell is unable to transport important nutrients. The amyloid precursor protein is cleaved by an enzyme called *alpha secretase*. This creates sticky abnormally folded protein chunks that impede communication between adjacent nerve cells. Isolated neurons eventually die in the hippocampus region impacting the person's ability to encode, store, and retrieve new memories (Durso et al. 2013).

While Alzheimer's is the most well-known type of dementia others exist as well. I fondly recall one of my dearest couples. I had the pleasure of caring for him after he presented with recurrent syncope, or passing out, at the dinner table. His wife was a devoted and committed caregiver. When we met, she was desperate for answers.

He was seen and treated by an electrophysiologist who specialized in the treatment of irregular heart rhythms. He was diagnosed with atrial fibrillation and received a pacemaker. He felt better but by the third month he was continued to have recurrent syncope. The drop attacks occurred at his dinner table and periodically while he attended church services.

This became a major source of stress and worry, both to the patient and to his devoted family. Putting on my geriatric cap, I decided it was time to delve much deeper into his geriatric assessment. When I asked Mr. X about his memory, he seemed quite unbothered. However, collateral history from his wife revealed some important nuggets. He was forgetting to organize his medications in the last eight to twelve months.

Mr. X typically enjoyed hunting outdoors with friends and frolicking with his grandchildren. In the last year before establishing care, she revealed that he was less engaged. He was sleeping more in the daytime and acting out his dreams. "I just thought you sleep more when you're tired, so I chalked it up to that!" She later went on to cinch the diagnosis when she started to recall how he was so preoccupied with talking to "these little kids." Mr. X reiterated her findings, stating that he was sleeping more but was delighted to see his grandkids more frequently.

This constellation of memory loss, visual hallucinations, and recurrent falls was classic for Lewy Body dementia. In this form of dementia, patients have fluctuating periods of alertness like Mr. X. Patients also have a defective protein called *alpha synuclein*. This protein also regulates the function of neurons in another region of the brain the controls movement. Lewy Body patients typically have overlapping features of Parkinsonism given their altered levels of dopamine.

This overlapping dependence on dopamine is the reason why geriatricians warn relatives to avoid giving antipsychotics to these patients for hallucinations. Antipsychotics like Haldol and Risperdal can deplete the supply of dopamine leading to a medical emergency called Neuroleptic malignant syndrome. In this condition, patients develop, fevers, rapid heart rate, and life-threatening muscle damage. The use of antipsychotics can also exacerbate the underlying memory disorder in Lewy Body. Knowing the diagnosis, we were able to provide reassurance about the visual hallucinations and recurrent falls. Mr. X was started on medications and lifestyle changes.

Lewy Body Dementia can be confused with Parkinson dementia. The caveat is that memory loss in Parkinsonian patients tends to follow motor dysfunction after many years. Conversely, in Lewy Body, motor instability may occur simultaneously with memory loss or within one to two years.

The other types of dementia include vascular dementia, which is functional memory loss that occurs following a stroke or cerebrovascular accident. Persons with blockages in the internal carotid arteries, the *pipes of the neck*, are prone to this form of dementia. Why, may you ask? The internal carotid arteries beautifully connect to the lush circle of blood vessels in the brain called the *circle of Willis*. Pieces of plaque and cholesterol can travel up the internal carotids directly in the ophthalmic artery causing temporary loss of vision. Portions of cholesterol can also escape and travel into the middle cerebral artery. This artery intricately supplies the terrain of the brain that is responsible for movement and speech.

Whatever the mechanism, be it pieces of plaque that embolize to parts of the brain or narrowing of the blood vessel walls from years of cholesterol accumulation, patients with strokes are at risk for cognitive decline following a stroke. Vascular dementia damages the cables or white matter nerve fibers that connect the memory centers. These white matter changes can be viewed nicely on imaging diffusion weighted MRIs of the brain. Seniors with vascular dementia can make memories, but they struggle to retrieve the memories due to changes in the white matter. These patients respond best to environmental cuing, such as lists and white boards.

As I pen this book, another dementia that has been discussed is a variant of Alzheimer's dementia called

TDP-43, named after the defective protein seen in autopsy in patients with memory loss. TDP-43 has been linked to dementia in the oldest seniors. In contrast to TDP-43, another classic dementia exists that all savvy seniors must know.

Two years ago, a fairly young sixty-year-old male came with his partner to establish care. His past medical history on the surface was remarkable, indicating only gastroesophageal reflux and occasional arthritis. He and his partner were planning a life together and were hoping to wed quite soon. In our initial visit, as we started our geriatric review of systems, the one that stood out completely was his eccentric behavior. He was having more difficulty navigating his car and had been in several fender benders. He was amenable to a non-renewal of his driving license.

His MOCA was less than 26, suggesting some level of impairment. The areas that were most affected were his ability to connect the trail dots and to draw a clock. As the history continued, the partner became more candid about his mood changes. "He'll just get so focused when we go walking but wouldn't want to listen to me, I tell him to be safe, but he just gets so agitated!" These phrases were like music to my ears. The history of behavioral changes, combined with poor executive function on the MOCA and his normal labs, suggested a frontotemporal dementia.

This type of dementia classically occurs in younger patients like the one described. There are two variants.

The first is the behavioral variant which the patient demonstrated. Patients become more restless, outspoken, hyperoral and may even become hypersexual. Treatment is focused on the behaviors. The second variant of fronto-temporal dementia is the language variant, where patients lose the ability to converse in a meaningful way. They may have problems with language production and language understanding. On an MRI, this patient had significant loss of the matter in the frontal and temporal regions of his brain.

Despite these common dementias, others exist. Some patients can develop functional memory loss from other conditions such as HIV or following long hospital critical illnesses. There is much discussion about the risks of developing a COVID-related dementia. Whatever the etiology, the unifying feature of any dementia is the association of cerebral domain impairment with an inability to function.

Geriatricians are trained to ensure that sexy and savvy seniors remain highly functional. Most geriatricians take a holistic approach to care. All my patients are educated about the MiND diet. This is the Mediterranean and Dash diet for neurodegenerative delay. This diet is based on the premise that the certain foods are inherently neuroprotective. Blueberries, blackberries, and strawberries contain a chemical called anthocyanin, which helps the cells in the hippocampus that are essential for memory. Nuts provide antioxidants that reduce cell damage in the brain. The MiND diet is rich is berries, nuts, and fish. This enables seniors to make healthier choices and limit the consumption of fried, starchy foods that are not as beneficial for their brain.

ARE THERE ANY COMMUNITIES WHERE THE PREVALENCE OF DEMENTIA IS LOW?

I would be remiss if I did not mention the blue zones. What are blue zones? I'm glad you asked. Nestled throughout the world are several regions that boast of centenarians with low rates of chronic disease. These regions were initially described by Italian internist Dr. Gianni Pes and Belgian astrophysicist Dr. Michel Poulain. In early 2000, both researchers identified several geographic regions where longevity is not the exception it is the norm. Over time, Dan Buettner, National Geographic journalist and bestselling author, garnered more attention for featuring these aging hotspots in the November 2005 edition of National Geographic. Before you leave this book to rush online to reserve your plane ticket there or rev up your google search engine, allow me the honor of being your virtual blue zone tour guide.

Blue zone communities exist in Okinawa, Japan, Sardinia, Italy, Nicoya, Costa Rica, Icaria, Greece, and among Seventh-day Adventists who reside in Loma Linda, California. These five regions share the distinct privilege of having residents who have only a fracture of the comorbidities that we battle so routinely in the Western world. What reduces their risk of developing cardiac disease, malignancies, and dementia? While you might be tempted to think it is impeccable genes or even preventative screening, blue zones share several key features. Residents live a life of purpose, they nurture social relationships, they are physically active, avoid tobacco use, and indulge in diets similar in composition to the MiND diet. Their diets are plant based and rich in vegetables and legumes.

CHAPTER 2

HOW SAVVY SENIORS
SELECT THEIR PHYSICIAN

Millions of seniors eagerly anticipate age sixty-five, when their red and white card is delivered in the mail confirming that they qualify for Medicare. Some patients are automatically enrolled while other patients must sign up during various annual enrollment periods. The first occurs from January through March while the latter occurs from October to December. During these periods, seniors shrewdly consult with their insurance companies to select the prescription drug plans, benefits, and physician groups best suited for their medical conditions.

Medicare is the health care coverage of approximately forty-six million seniors and nine million younger adults with disabilities. It was incepted in 1965 by then President Lynden Johnson. Through its component parts, A, B, and D, it provides coverage for acute hospitalizations, ambulatory preventative clinic visits, post-acute care, and prescription medications. As Altman and Frist describe, Medicare signaled an important step in the onerous journey for Civil rights for African Americans. Medicare helped to desegregate many hospitals that did not accept or manage minorities (Altman and Frist 2015).

With the passage of the Social Security Amendments of 1965, Medicare health coverage was established for persons over sixty-five, while Medicaid was launched for persons under the financial poverty line. Over the last five decades both coverages have undergone major revisions.

The business of Medicare and Medicaid remains a polarizing issue not only for obvious health related reasons but because it significantly impacts the bottom line of the US economy. Medicare accounts for approximately 14 percent of the federal budget. Medicare beneficiaries recognize this and consistently rank Medicare as one of the key issues they focus on when casting their votes in US primary and general elections.

It is often said that's a nation's health is its wealth. Once disparities in health care are eliminated, patients can focus their energies on obtaining the best physician for them. Each time I sit down with a patient for their initial clinic visit, I always start with one critical question. How did you hear about our practice? I have noticed two major categories of answers.

Some patients take a more passive approach in their selection. They were randomly assigned to the practice by their insurance company or on the recommendation of a trusted friend. The second group is more proactive and intentional about their selection. These bosses have done their homework. They have searched for the practice online. They have meticulously read the google reviews of the clinic and providers. They have paid close attention to the physician's medical and postgraduate certification.

No two patients are alike. However, I can almost guarantee that the patients who follow the *Age Like Royalty Roadmap* are very intentional with how they select their medical provider. These savvy and sassy seniors also seem to operate with the principle of the three A's. Regardless of race, ethnicity, creed, or gender, they desire a physician who is affable, able, and available. Why didn't I mention affordable? Well, if a practice demonstrates the three As, patients are eager and happy to compensate the physician for their time and expertise. You know what else? They will share their treasured prize with other likeminded individuals who want the same outcomes in their medical care.

My enthusiastic internal medicine residency program director, Dr. Manthous, and my unforgettable ambulatory Attending Dr. Manisha Gupta both stressed that the best physicians are not the smartest physicians but simply the ones who are truly invested in their patients. They take the time to listen to their patients, meticulously gather and peruse prior medical records. I continue to stress this to my medical residents when I precept them on hospital rounds. I also remind them that the best doctors demonstrate a level of professionalism, empathy, and bedside rapport that is authentic. They establish a relationship with patients that does not encroach on personal boundaries but one where the lines of communication remain open.

Exemplary physicians embody these attributes and encourage it in their colleagues. They recognize that in a time of telemedicine, savvy seniors have a diverse option of physicians to choose from. I cannot tell you how often exasperated patients exclaim, "My old doctor was an exceptional physician, but his/her staff was just plain rude and disorganized, and there's no way I'm going back!"

Savvy seniors need and deserve a medical practice where everyone has a proverbial horse in the race. As I alluded to in an earlier chapter, each member, from the transportation driver to the receptionist, medical assistant, pharmacist, and practitioner, must realize their role in creating a world-class experience for each patient. Patients must not be regarded as another number. The practices that provide stellar senior care refuse to settle for mediocrity, have zero tolerance for unprofessionalism, and are committed to partnering with their clients to address the medical, spiritual, psychological, and functional aspects of their care.

Many families typically have a family physician who cares for the entire clan. This person is highly treasured in the community. Word of mouth testimonial referrals are perhaps still the best for a budding physician who is establishing their brand and reputation. If a patient has received exemplary care in the hospital from an internist, the chances are extremely high that they will pursue ongoing outpatient care following discharge. The bond between the patient and physician can become so strong that many patients will keep their internist well into their prime.

THE POWER OF LISTENING

"You were the first person who took the time to listen, you actually listened to me!" I cannot tell you how the art of silence is so treasured by a savvy senior. I see my patients' lives as a complex novel with intricate details. Often because of our fast-paced society, many patients feel that the essence of their story may not be captured in a fifteen-minute quota of time. Fearing that the doctor will not get to truly hear them, some approach an initial visit with a barrage of questions and concerns that can leave a physician with more questions than answers. Others become frustrated when even a well-intentioned physician may trivialize, compartmentalize, or negate their presenting complaints.

I remember one such family who presented for a new patient encounter. The patient was an impeccably adorned Hispanic female in her mid-seventies. Polished and well groomed, her fingernails were coated with beautiful pink polish that matched the rose color of her face mask. Immediately, I could tell she was fiercely independent.

She was accompanied by her daughter, her doppelganger, who was her caregiver. The daughter was highly organized. She had a carrier with her mother's medication and discharge paperwork. She had a separate lunch kit with a snack and her mother's daytime insulin.

As I walked in to garner the history, the patient's warm hazel eyes greeted me over her face shield. I interrogated the patient about her previous hospitalization but my attempts to engage the daughter proved less successful since she was laser focused on reviewing the paperwork. I whispered a quick prayer, drew closer, sat my clipboard down, and humbly asked, "Can you please tell me your story in your very own words?"

I listened intently as she recounted the night, she woke up gasping for air. Her husband frantically dialed 911. She was admitted and diuresed. She was later discharged to a skilled nursing facility for short-term rehab. She mustered up the grit Sylvester Stallone displayed in his Rocky Balboa franchise to complete rehab as soon as possible to reunite with her love of forty years!

She continued with outpatient physical therapy where she had her near-death experience. "I was doing my exercises and just when I went to turn around with my walker, I felt dizzy and nauseous, I told the therapist I'm going to faint!" The therapist calmly sat her down and immediately beckoned her daughter who was waiting in the lobby.

The daughter then interjected and continued the story. With adrenaline racing, she helped her mom to the car and sped to the Emergency room. I could see the tears welling in her eyes. During the ride, she kept talking to her mother. "Doctor, that day I thought I was going to lose my mom forever!"

I was magnetically entrenched in every detail of the story. I interjected only for minor clarification and to add an assuring nod to show that I had grasped the severity of this harrowing ER event. The story easily rivalled any riveting Hollywood blockbuster. The patient eventually had to have immediate transvenous cardiac pacemaker placement right in the emergency room because her pulse became dangerously low.

The patient suffered an acute myocardial infarction of her right coronary vessel. This vessel receives its innervation from the same nerve that innervates the gastric system. This explained her nausea at the therapist's office. The right coronary artery supplies blood to the pacemaker region of the heart that sets the speed of the heart rate. Ischemia (inadequate blood supply) in the right coronary can result in symptomatic and fatal bradycardia.

Sitting there and listening allowed the patient and her daughter to be validated. It enabled us to craft a plan that addressed each of the patient's medical issues. It provided us time to successfully reconcile her hospital discharge medications. Despite having to move on to another patient, the patient and her daughter had no qualms about staying behind until the close of the clinic to ensure that all their concerns were addressed.

As a physician to my senior gems, I see this story exemplified in my younger patients as well. Like Dr. William Osler stated, the patient already knows his or her diagnosis. He or she only needs us to translate that layman's diagnosis into formal medical jargon. Seniors who follow the *Age Like Royalty Roadmap* seek out physicians who are knowledgeable and who will listen. I treasure the adage, patients don't care how much you know, until they know how much you care! Sitting and listening in a non-judgmental way guarantees that the physician will get the maximum results of their history taking.

CHAPTER 3

——•——

WHY SAVVY SENIORS NEED A GERIATRICIAN

The population of savvy seniors is soaring is due to important medical advancements including vaccinations, preventive health screenings, and lifelong management of comorbid diseases. It is estimated that in less than forty years, one in four persons will be over the age of sixty-five in the United States. Savvy seniors, and in some cases, their children, typically have many questions and concerns about the impact of aging on their health. In much the same way that a new mother would carefully enlist the expertise and skill of a neonatal pediatrician, savvy seniors are focused on ensuring that their nuanced questions about aging will be answered by internists who are trained in this field.

One of my dearest patients is a well-versed, highly functioning octogenarian. Mrs. G reads daily, exercises, astutely manages her finances, and keeps abreast with the modern advances in medicine. "I was scouring on google to find a doctor for seniors, and then I came across you!" Intrigued about what motivated her search, I asked her to elaborate as I pulled up a seat to listen. She confided in me that she had been seeing her primary care doctor for four decades. Albeit she had received her annual age-appropriate vaccines and yearly physicals, something was still lacking. She had a cabinet full of nutraceuticals and over-the-counter vitamins that could rival any pharmacy. Every year it seemed like another medication and herbal supplement had been added to her burgeoning list of medications.

Mrs. G was a sassy and savvy senior who demanded change. She wanted to reap the benefits of all of her years of hard labor. She wished to not only survive but thrive during her retirement years. She wanted to actively learn about the conditions that were germane to aging so she could better understand the geriatric syndromes for which she was at risk such as falls. Mrs. G desired a physician who provided only essential medications and explained the rationale behind the medication selection.

She wanted more from her healthcare provider, and she was determined to get it. She wanted a partnership where she was an equal stakeholder, and her perspective was solicited in the creation of her care plan. The thing that I remember the most about her quest for a geriatrician was the last thing she told me. "Dr. Rodgers, I have been seeing my practitioner for close to forty years, but I can't guarantee that if we were to meet on the street, he'd even know my name!" Mrs. G took the bold step to find the doctor for her and unapologetically never looked back. We have embarked on an amazing journey that continues to this day.

Ms. J, twenty years her junior, had worked in accounting for years as a supervisor. Her daughter lived outside the state but started to realize that something was wrong when Ms. J missed several rental payments and was close to eviction. Concerned that an even greater memory issue could be looming, she enlisted the help of a geriatrician.

WHAT IS A GERIATRICIAN?

Geriatrics is the branch of medicine devoted to the care of seniors. It was first coined in 1891 and derives its name from *geron,* the Greek word for old. Gerontology is focused on the research that goes into aging. Geriatrics is the field that focuses on the medical management of persons over sixty-five. Like cardiology or pediatrics, Geriatrics is a distinct subspecialty. Medical doctors termed *fellows* apply to study geriatrics after completing four years of medical school and three years of internal medicine residency training.

Several geriatric programs exist in the United States. The programs span one to two years. In the first-year, medical fellows manage patients in a wide array of settings. These include hospital wards, long term care units, rehabilitation facilities, adult day programs or Program of All-inclusive care of the Elderly (PACE), and ambulatory offices. They even manage patients in the comfort of their own homes. This training is even more timely in the COVID-19 era in which we live. Geriatric fellows who complete a second year typically use the additional twelve months to finalize and present geriatric-centered research.

With our aging gems shining brighter and longer, the demand for geriatricians is at its all-time highest. JoAnn Jenkins, the CEO of AARP, sounded the alarm of the geriatrician shortage in her 2016 best seller *Disrupt Aging*. She indicated that only eleven of 145 medical schools in the United States have departments of geriatric medicine. Mrs. Johnson revealed the harsh reality that fewer than 1 percent of nurses are geriatric trained.

Medical schools and medical residencies have heard the clarion call for greater teaching of geriatrics. They have responded by introducing geriatric courses into their curricula quite early. This move is beneficial for two reasons. It equips students with the principles needed to master care for seniors in the inpatient, long term care, and ambulatory settings. It exposes these brilliant minds to the field of geriatrics in the hopes that they will one day also eventually pursue it.

At the time that *Disrupt Aging* was published in 2016, the US had approximately seven thousand board certified geriatricians. This translated to one geriatrician providing care for every two thousand Americans over age seventy-five. Because of these startling statistics, many savvy seniors have begun to actively seek out their services. But you may be asking, "What makes this endangered group of specialists so unique?" In other words, what does a geriatrician offer that my primary care provider doesn't (Jenkins 2016).

IT'S ALL ABOUT THE FUNCTION!

If you are reading this book, clearly you are in an elite group of seniors who are intentional about being the boss of their aging. Geriatricians are guided by the desire to maintain our patients' independence and function for as long as humanly possible. After establishing rapport with their patients, they craft a customized treatment plan and see their patients as often as it takes to identify and successfully manage their issues. Geriatrics is a team player specialty. We believe in the power of interdisciplinary care. Hence, geriatricians like myself work hand-in-hand with nurses, pharmacists, psychiatrists, physical therapists, etc. to maximize our patients' outcomes. Along with understanding the biology and pathophysiology of aging, geriatricians not only know how to treat the disease but how to treat the patient with the disease. Seniors present so differently that all geriatricians know that if you have treated one senior, you have only treated one senior.

WHAT CARE CAN YOU EXPECT FROM YOUR GERIATRICIAN?

Geriatricians are a unique breed of physicians. We are observant and often unassuming. We absolutely enjoy our patients so much so that we literally watch your every move. As I am writing this book, I am watching my mother as she happily sashays around my childhood home in the Bahamas. She is oblivious to the fact that I am analyzing her gait speed, stride length, and body posturing just to name a few. Why? Well, these simple observations can clue my sister onto the future potential for falls.

When savvy seniors arrive for their geriatric visits, they know they will receive the royal treatment. Geriatricians use the 5M technique to comprehensively assess their patients. This technique is utilized by the Canadian and American Geriatrics Societies. The first M is the more traditional review of multiplexity. Geriatricians review the treatment plans for their patient's chronic diseases. They ensure their vitals are reaching their goals and their laboratory values are appropriate. We will discuss these targets in a later chapter.

In the second M, geriatricians explore the mobility challenges of their patients. We enquire about falls, the fear of falling and possible fall risks. Like I alluded to with my mother, we use simple in office techniques like the timed up and go test. The physician analyzes the patient as they rise from a seated chair with no arm rests. The patient walks ten feet and returns to the chair. The patient is instructed to walk normally. They can use their assistive device if needed. The physician measures the time in seconds that it takes to rise, walk, and return to the chair.

Patients who require more than twelve seconds typically have associated muscle wasting and balance issues. Once determined, the geriatrician can immediately make recommendations for interventions such as outpatient physical strengthening geared at muscle strengthening and balance. They can also determine if a patient may benefit from an assistive device like a single-point or tripod cane or rollator walker.

The third M is geared at examining the patient's mind and mood. After taking a thorough medical, social, and family history from their patients, geriatricians perform mental and mood assessments. The Mini-cog is used to screen for the presence of memory impairment. It is one of my favorites. During the test, the examiner repeats three words. The patient must commit the words to memory. Once this is done the examiner instructs the patient to draw a clock depicting a specific time. All clocks and watches are removed from the patient's field of view. Following the clock draw the examiner asks the patient to recite the original three words. The Mini-cog is scored out of five points. Two points are given if the clock is circular, the numbers are well-spaced, and the time depicted is correct. Three additional points are given if all three words are correctly recited. Geriatricians pursue further memory testing using a MOCA test if a patient has an incorrect clock and recalls only one of three words. The test is also concerning if the word recall is also zero.

The most common test to screen for depression is the geriatric depression screen or GDS. This test differs from the popular PHQ-9. Both tests can be used in the mood assessment of seniors. In fact, the PHQ-9 has a reasonable sensitivity and specificity depression screening. The GDS is customized for seniors because the questions focus more on the senior's emotional well-being. The PHQ-9 asks questions about problems with sleep, appetite, and energy. These vague questions may be confounded by other comorbidities in aging. A senior with respiratory failure may score high for depression using the PHQ-9 based on somatic symptoms that are due primarily from their COPD.

During the GDS, the patient is asked fifteen questions about their emotional health. Questions include their preferences about going out to socialize or staying inside along with their perception on whether they are happy to be alive right now. These questions are more streamlined to focus on their mental well-being. A patient who scores over 5 on the GDS raises flags for depression.

The fourth M is huge in the world of geriatrics. It is medication. Geriatricians not only review medication lists, but they also identify barriers for proper compliance such as lack of a pill box or confusion with the pills. They also determine if the mode of medication delivery needs to be adjusted. Patients with severe degenerative arthritis will need to have pill bottle caps that are less cumbersome to open. In the past, I have changed my patients' medications to pre-sorted pill packs to reduce the risk of exceeding the intended dose.

The average person over sixty-five meets criteria for polypharmacy. They have at least five more drugs on their medication list. The adverse drug reactions from polypharmacy accounts for nearly 25 percent of all senior visits to the emergency room. There is hope, however, and we can stem this tide. Geriatricians are trained specifically to review medication lists at each visit. The prescribing cascade occurs where a drug is given by a well-meaning provider to treat the side effects of another medication. For example, the patient is prescribed a diuretic after developing swollen ankles. The patient and provider may unknowingly fail to recognize that an antihypertensive like amlodipine may be the culprit of the swollen ankles. Simply switching to another antihypertensive class can avert expanding the medication list. Geriatricians like myself always enquire and review the medication list when a patient has a new presenting complaint. We also take the time to discuss the use of over-the-counter medications, nutraceuticals, herbal teas, and bush medicines, just to name a few. My patients and I get excited when we find ways to shrink their medicine list.

Taking the time to do a careful medication reconciliation can avert an adverse drug effect that can lead to a preventable hospitalization and even death. Geriatricians review high risk medications like insulin, opioids, and benzodiazepines. They take the extra time to ensure they are abiding by the guiding principles of the Beers list when they prescribe a new medication. They are on high alert for dangerous drug-drug interactions. One of my dear sassy and savvy patients takes comfort in having a geriatrician simply because she is assured that I will inform her cardiologists about any medications that can have untoward side-effects. This interdisciplinary approach maximizes outcomes.

The final M that geriatricians assess is what matters most to their patients. I know what you're thinking. She's about to talk about end of life, advanced planning, wills. Yes, I will do that in a later chapter, but I am focused on what matters most in a patient's day to day life. These goals may include being able to keep their driver's license. It may include being able to navigate social media to communicate with loved ones during COVID-19. I like to consider myself their fairy goal mother. I get to use creativity and work with their families to maintain their function and independence.

HOW DOES A GERIATRICIAN DIAGNOSE DIFFERENTLY?

By now, I trust that you are seeing that geriatricians are physicians who manage complex conditions. They distinguish themselves, however, by taking a step back from the patient to manage their patients holistically. Geriatricians want their patients to boss up. To do that, they identify conditions that other specialists may unknowingly ignore. These conditions are collectively termed geriatric syndromes. They are the bread and butter of geriatric medicine.

Geriatric syndromes that are unrecognized and untreated increase the risk of hospitalization and death. While the cardiologist focuses on congestive heart failure or the pulmonologist hones in on chronic obstructive pulmonary disease (COPD), geriatricians are lasered in on detecting syndromes that include falls, polypharmacy, dementia, incontinence, depression, malnutrition, etc. (Ouslander 2018).

A geriatric syndrome is a complex multifactorial condition that can have grave effects on a senior's quality of life. These syndromes can increase the rate that a person deteriorates from their ongoing chronic comorbidities. Let me illustrate this point. Doctors classify the functional severity of heart failure using the New York Heart Association Functional Classification system. Persons at Stage 1 experience symptoms on maximal exertion like running a marathon while a person at Stage II may become symptomatic as he or she performs house chores. Patients at Stage III report symptoms with minimal activity and Stage IV patients experience symptoms at rest. Let's suppose that Mr. J and Mr. K both have New York Functional

Stage III Heart failure. They are both only able to perform simple activities of daily living, like bathing, before becoming winded. Suppose that they both share a diagnosis of insomnia and depression and are managed with a selective serotonin inhibitor (SSRI) such as Citalopram.

Let's postulate even further. Mr. J's non-geriatric physician, though well-meaning, prescribes Ambien to help the patient with bouts of insomnia. Mr. K's geriatrician recognizes the physiologic changes of aging and the potential for falls. He explains his concerns to Mr. K. Together, they opt to increase the dose of the citalopram and start cognitive behavioral therapy.

Mr. J, in contrast, is started on Ambien, and as time goes on the doses are never weaned. As I stated earlier in this chapter, due to changes in physiology, he is relatively sedated and sustains a fall on the way to the bathroom. This results in a hip fracture leading to a hospitalization and rehabilitation. He is immobilized and develops a decubitus ulcer that becomes infected at rehabilitation. The infection spreads to his bloodstream causing septicemia. This exacerbates his underlying congestive cardiac failure and Mr. J spirals on a downward trajectory. This case is fictional, but it can occur in real life. It can be avoided when physicians partner with geriatricians who understand the principle pharmacologic and physiologic changes that occur with aging.

CHAPTER 4

ASSEMBLING THE ROYAL COURT: KEY PARTNERSHIPS AS YOU AGE

In September 2019, I returned to the Bahamas exactly twenty-four hours before the catastrophic landfall of the deadliest hurricane in my nation's history. Hurricane Dorian, a Category 5 phenom, decimated the beautiful islands of Abaco and Grand Bahama in ways that were unimaginable. Hundreds of families recounted the harrowing tales of the moment their loved ones perished. No one in the country, myself included, was exempt. Hurricane Dorian left its devastating imprint on everyone for decades to come.

In the aftermath of Dorian, I had time to reflect on my life and its true purpose. In a surreal turn of events, God allowed me to cross paths with Medical Mogul, entrepreneur, and life coach Dr. Draion Burch. Through his high-energy and upbeat persona, he forced me to re-examine the goals I had set for my life. More importantly, he challenged me to identify the muse behind my drive. After days of prayer, it was clear that my why was my family.

Like so many others, my parents sacrificed so much for me on my journey through medicine. Whether it be by giving sound advice, or by taking incessant collect charges in the pre-cell phone era, Hermon and Sylvia Rodgers continue to remain my staunch supporters through all the stages of medicine. Yet, as I watch my parents navigate their own aging process, I realize that they could not thrive without the unwavering support of their own caregiving team chaired by my sister.

My sister never asked for this duty, but she embraced it with enviable grace and poise. She is the caregiver that I wish all my patients could have. I often ask, why do you do it? She simply responds in her direct matter of fact tone, "The Bible says honoring your father and mother is what you do, and I am happy that I can do it!"

SELECTING A CAREGIVER

Caregiving is an art that few will master with such precision as my sister. She often jokes that she was often terrified of older people when she was a little girl, but she has now developed a reverential admiration for them. She sees them through a completely different lens. I want to say that having a baby sister as an internist and geriatrician has mellowed her, but I recognize that she is successful at caregiving because she has three key innate skills. She is methodical, meticulous about details, and is a fearless advocate for our parents.

Kathrina always ensures that I am kept abreast of any changes in disposition. She and my brother-in-law, Ralph, help to coordinate doctors' visits. She ensures that medication refills are done in a timely manner and is a voracious reader who stays abreast of all pertinent geriatric issues. At the onset of COVID-19, she ordered several massage devices that my parents used to substitute for outpatient physical therapy. This initiative ensured they would stay active at home as they quarantined.

As a geriatrician, I have had the pleasure of meeting other caregivers with the same passion for providing excellent care. One male caregiver, Ravi, whom I still communicate with to this day, did an exceptional job with his mother. He carefully researched and hired skilled home attendants for her personal care and familiarized himself with his mother's appropriate geriatric syndromes. More importantly, he continued to advocate for his mother through every procedure and hospitalization. This ensured that she received appropriate levels of care.

It is estimated that there are approximately forty million caregivers in the US. These unsung heroes are the wind beneath my patients' wings. Sassy and savvy seniors are intentional when they assemble their royal court. They select caregivers that are reliable, consistent, and truly invested in their care. They identify these individuals years before there is an unexpected medical emergency. They are the ones that accompany their relatives to the doctor's office. They are trusted to weigh in on important medical decisions such as medications and surgical interventions. Their invaluable service is often neglected. Unfortunately, they too can face the harsh realities of life if they do not take time to recharge themselves.

I always recommend that my sassy and savvy seniors select more than one caregiver. It may be an offspring, sibling, trusted friend, or neighbor. Caregivers should communicate regularly and can delegate specific tasks. The primary caregiver may assist with managing health and finance related issues. The secondary caregiver may be solely responsible for completing pharmacy and grocery store errands. Why do you need to assemble a royal court as you age? Depending on one sole caregiver can become perilous if that person is suddenly incapacitated and unable to continue the role. Sole caregivers can also develop debilitating challenges in the process.

Caregiver fatigue is the term used to describe the stress and symptomology many caregivers experience as they grapple with caring for a loved one with multiple co-morbidities. Caregivers can find that their own health deteriorates. They may develop hypertension or suboptimal diabetes control. The grueling physical effects of helping their loved ones with activities of daily living like bathing and dressing can result in pain or stiffness such as osteo-arthritic back pain. Research has shown that caregivers have an increased chance of developing psychological issues. They are more prone to anxiety and depression (Ouslander 2018).

Geriatricians and internists who care for sassy and savvy seniors must take time to explore the mental and physical health of their patient's caregiver. I always include caregivers in the development of my management plan as they are the pivotal in ensuring that the details are executed. Caregivers are the quarterbacks in the game of aging.

Before COVID and the global launch of telemedicine, I always made it my priority to speak to my patient's caregiver via speaker phone, WhatsApp, or via email. The reason for this communication was twofold. It ensured that the essence and key pearls of the management plan were communicated clearly to the family. More importantly, it allowed me to check in with the caregiver to determine how the disease process was affecting their quality of life. All my caregivers appreciated this extra personalized human touch. I truly believe it further deepened our trust and rapport.

I would be remiss if I did not take the time to acknowledge caregivers like Ravi and my sister, Kathrina. They took up the mantle of caregiving with unspeakable grace. These unsung heroes have a level of grit and resilience that is unmatched. If you are or know someone who is a caregiver, please take the opportunity to acknowledge their exceptional love and service. I always remind caregivers like my sister to take time out for self-care. This may come in the form of going on a vacation, going to the spa for a day of pampering, going for a walk, or simply taking time to listen to soothing music. We all need to find that happy place where we can retreat and rejuvenate.

The other piece in the royal armamentarium of savvy seniors is their spiritual ethos. Faith remains a key cornerstone in the fabric of their existence. They have some spiritual foundation that enables them to cope with the vicissitudes of life. They faithfully subscribe to a daily routine where uninterrupted time is carved out for prayer, reflection, and meditation. During these moments of solitude, they can be vulnerable and honestly face their fears. These scheduled escapades are undisturbed by the incessant clamor of cell phones, the screams of grandkids, or the audible vibrato of texts. Savvy seniors emerge revitalized with the motivation needed to age with poise.

Savvy seniors understand that no man is an island. Their social circles dwindle as they suffer the sometimes-unexpected loss of confidantes, lovers, and even children. Nevertheless, they maintain quality friendships. Their intimate circles are filled with people with whom they can share the realities of aging. They include persons with similar interests like playing golf, gardening, watching soap operas, and mentoring. Communal relationships were affected significantly during COVID-19. Many community groups disbanded or converted their meetings to an online platform. Seniors who were unable to attend virtually were faced with even greater feelings of isolation and depression.

Partnerships are essential on the road to aging like royalty. Savvy seniors build partnerships with organizations that focus on their financial and legal affairs. They are knowledgeable about the agencies on elder law and aging in their community. They are educated and well-versed on governmental policies that impact their health care and retirement. They seek out information about agencies who provide meaningful services such as meal delivery and transportation.

On the yellow brick road to aging with dignity, savvy seniors always make a purposeful detour to review their financial outlook. They invest in getting all the legal information they need to conduct proper estate planning. So many celebrities with massive amounts of wealth pass away with no estate planning. So many seniors die unexpectedly, leaving their families unable to cover their medical or burial expenses. Why? They often neglected their finances thinking they would eventually get around to it.

Savvy seniors avoid procrastination. They enlist the aid of a professional financial and estate planner early on. They itemize their physical and non-physical assets such as insurance policies and bank accounts. They detail their expenses. They designate transfer of beneficiaries on death and make provisions for all heirs, including pets. They appoint a trusted and competent executor of their estate. On a practical level, they make copies of their legal wills and regularly revise the will after any significant life events.

CHAPTER 5

LEAVING A LASTING
HONORABLE LEGACY

End-of-life discussions create perhaps the greatest amounts of anxiety and angst in patients and, yes, even doctors. Though we may deny it, few people are excited to spend their waking moments planning their final days. This is usually an afterthought in young adulthood. Many young people are preoccupied with immortality and believe that they will stay forever young.

As a geriatrician, I have seen a paradigm shift in the minds of savvy seniors. These patients recognize the complexities and intricacies of life. They understand how fragile life is. They may have experienced unexpected tragedies in their families. Many are convinced that they do not want to be a financial or physical burden on their loved ones. They take financial planning for retirement as seriously as medical planning for end of life.

If you're reading this book, you may know someone who has been confronted with the question, "Do you want us to do everything?" This is question that is asked by a well-meaning ER or hospitalist physician in the wake of a life-shattering emergency such as a heart attack or myocardial infarction. Savvy seniors and their loved ones are fully prepared for this question. They have invested the time and energy in having these pivotal conversations in a relaxed environment before a devastating event.

Their geriatrician has introduced advanced care planning in a thoughtful manner. Patients are given brochures for advanced directives, such as the Five Wishes. This document allows seniors to meticulously outline their medical, personal, spiritual, and emotional needs at the end of life. I encourage my patients to complete their Five Wishes and review it with their relatives before it is witnessed and submitted. If they are hospitalized or treated in the ER, the Five Wishes can be revised and updated.

So, what are advanced directives? Advanced directives are a set of instructions that are discussed during advanced care planning. First, they allow seniors to delegate a medical proxy or medical power of attorney. The power of attorney can make medical decisions on the patient's behalf when the patient is unable to do so. The durable power of attorney can enact this right at any time. Patients are advised to select the person whom they feel will act in their best interests and execute their wishes if a terminal event arises. While many select their spouses or children, others may appoint a trusted friend.

The second decision that patients must make relates to their desire for resuscitation in the wake of sudden cardiac or respiratory arrest. Hollywood has sensationalized this process through the adrenaline surging depictions of defibrillation. Many patients are well acquainted with the resuscitation events captured by actors and actresses on television shows such as *ER* and *Grey's Anatomy*. An observational study done over three decades ago revealed that nearly 60 percent of patients over seventy form their opinion about CPR from television media. These depictions though do not always show the harrowing aftermath and consequences in the aged. These include fractured ribs, less than a five percent chance of survival, and ventilator dependence leading to the insertion of artificial airways and gastric devices. These are termed tracheostomy and percutaneous endoscopic gastrostomy (PEG) tubes (Semmens 2019).

Because they have both taken the time to invest in a deeper meaningful dialogue, savvy seniors and their doctors have specific and individualized goals of care. Some want to pursue longevity at all costs while others want to maintain a good quality of life. The latter will usually forego resuscitation if success leaves them immobile or unable to function independently.

Whatever the decision, savvy seniors are planners. They appreciate doctors who respect and honor their decisions but provide them with honest feedback on their prognosis. This enables them to make informed choices about the medical care they elect at the end of life.

PART 2:

THE ROYAL
SECRETS OF
LONGEVITY

CHAPTER 6

GERIATRICIAN/PATIENT RELATIONSHIP

As I write this book, the US Preventative task force has just reduced the initial age for screening colonoscopies from fifty to forty-five. This was done after it was determined that a large population of colon cancers were being diagnosed at a later stage. The need for preventative testing is a common question that patients over sixty-five ask their doctors. Many ageist myths out there lead many patients and families to forego justifiable medical treatments due to age. "I'm too old for that surgery, if they cut me, I won't make if off the table!" This is a popular sentiment that many patients and families express when confronted with different management plans.

Savvy seniors want physicians who recognize the difference between their patient's chronologic and physiologic age. Chronos or time refers to the patient's actual age while physiologic age is based on the patient's functional ability.

A healthy, fit octogenarian (eighty or older) with only hypertension, who can walk a mile daily, for example, cannot be viewed in the same vein as a sixty-nine-year-old with heart failure and diabetes. The human body does undergo changes with aging as discussed. There is diminished functional reserve in the organ systems. However, the patient's appropriateness for surgery or other management strategies such as chemotherapy must be determined on a case-by-case basis. This decision must balance the risk of the intervention with the suitability of the patient to withstand the intervention and benefit of the treatment.

Determining the course of action must also be based on the patient's understanding of their disease process and their ability to provide *informed consent.* During an informed consent, the patient must be able to communicate the benefit of the procedure and to express the consequences of no intervention at all. Informed consent involves the ability to reason with the information provided and to express an opinion that demonstrates a reasonable appreciation of the case.

Geriatricians help patients to ensure that their treatment goals are in line with their overall goals for health. This was the key component of the comprehensive geriatric assessment we discussed in Chapter 3. Competent geriatricians make the distinction between physiologic and chronologic age by conducting screening questions, tests, and physical examinations. These examinations collectively comprise the comprehensive geriatric assessment. As you may know, during a history the physician asks about past medical diagnoses, hospitalization, surgeries, and allergies. They delve into family history to determine a patient's risk of developing a disease. They enquire about the patient's immunization or vaccine history.

Physicians with a geriatric focus also discuss important issues that are germane to aging. These include a history of falls, memory loss, incontinence, sleep, driving difficulty, sensory loss such as hearing and vision, nutrition, and use of dentures. These topics are several important geriatric syndromes. Identification of these syndromes can help seniors more easily navigate the sometimes choppy tides of aging. To create a full masterpiece of their patient, they take time to address plans for end of life, proxies, or decision makers. Competent geriatricians ensure that the visits are not rushed so that they can capture the true essence of the patient whom they are privileged to care for.

CHAPTER 7

THERE'S NO PLACE LIKE HOME: PREVENTING HOSPITALIZATIONS

I have noticed several things that savvy seniors actively do to avoid hospitalizations. First, they select an affable, able, and available geriatrician with whom they have great rapport. They keep their appointments and avoid no-shows. Cancellations are almost non-existent and only occur in extraneous circumstances. They contact the office with well thought-out questions only if they are unable to get the answers for themselves.

Meticulous record-keeping is a key characteristic of savvy seniors. They keep updated logs of appropriate family history or genetic conditions if needed. They keep impeccable dates of all interactions with the healthcare system. These can range from visits to urgent care, elective surgeries, and past hospitalizations. They notate the findings of all imaging studies like MRIs or CAT Scans. Test results and hospital records are treasures if they are ever admitted to a hospital.

Savvy seniors are laser-focused on living their best lives. They value routine physical activity. They know that a body in motion should stay in motion. While many re-treated to their homes during COVID-19, sassy seniors engaged in gardening, walking their pets, or home exercises at least thirty minutes daily. Many know the secret to getting a heart-stomping workout is a pulse rate that is equal to 220 minus their age.

Along with physical activity and consuming healthy servings of fruit and vegetables, savvy seniors stay mentally agile. Grandfluencers (web-savvy seniors) are utilizing social media to stay connected to peers with similar passions. They are active on dating apps like *Our Time,* so getting admitted to the hospital is the last thing on their agenda. They are too busy expanding their social circles and ensuring that along with diet and exercise they are keeping up with their preventative screens.

Age fifty heralds the start of many preventative screens such as mammograms, according to the United States Preventative Task Force guideline. In October 2020, this governing body announced that they had changed the age of initial colonoscopy from fifty to forty-five. This is presumably to detect more abnormalities before they progress to advanced malignancies. Readers may remember hearing about the tragic passing of promising Hollywood actor Chadwick Boseman on multiple media outlets. He succumbed to stage 3 colonic carcinoma at age forty-three on August 28, 2020.

At age sixty-five, discussions begin about receiving the quadrivalent (four flu strains), high-dose Fluzone vaccine, and the Pneumovax 23 vaccine that protects against the twenty-three strains of bacterial causing pneumonia. Pneumovax is administered to all patients between the ages of nineteen and sixty-four with medical conditions like heart or lung disease and tobacco use. The shot is repeated in five years if the patient is immunocompromised. At sixty-five, patients get their final Pneumococcal vaccine. Prevnar 13 vaccine is usually administered one year before the Pneumovax 23. Both shots must be separated by a minimum of eight weeks. Immunocompromised patients over sixty-five can receive the vaccine again.

At the time of publishing this book, I am pleased to say several vaccines were approved for COVID-19 including: Moderna, Pfizer, Astra Zeneca, and Johnson and Johnson. There is also growing work into the development of a new COVID-19 oral pill. Many savvy seniors are concerned about the potential side effects of the COVID-19 vaccine. They respectfully discuss this with trusted medical providers to make the most informed decision for them.

Another vaccine that is administered at age fifty is the shingles vaccine. This vaccine is used to reduce the pain that results from herpes zoster, the virus responsible for chicken pox. Zoster nestles comfortably alongside the nerve endings called dermatomes. It re-emerges during periods of stress, illness, or fatigue. Outbreaks are characterized by blisters in a linear dermatomal pattern. If the virus infects nerve endings in the tip of the nose, the Hutchinson's signature rash ensues. This is an ophthalmologic emergency because it can lead to painful vision loss.

The antidote is an oral antiviral like acyclovir for seven days and a topical cream for the intense neuropathic burning. This burning is called post herpetic neuralgia and its occurrence is reduced by administering two doses of the shingles vaccine six months apart.

For women over sixty-five, pap smears end if they had three normal smears in the preceding ten years. The last normal pap smear should be within the past five years. Seniors who are current smokers or those who quit in the last fifteen years get an annual low dose CT screening of the lungs if they have at least twenty "pack years" of tobacco use. These scans are reimbursed by insurance companies starting from age fifty-five to seventy-five. Men between sixty-five and seventy-five who have smoked more than 100 cigarettes in their entire lifetime get a one-time abdominal aortic ultrasound. This detects potentially fatal aortic aneurysms over four centimeters wide.

Another important screening measure for women is the dual energy X-ray absorptiometry, or DEXA, which assesses the bone mineral density of bones in the lumbar spine, hip, or femoral, and radial forearm. Postmenopausal women have accelerated bone loss due to estrogen decline. A surrogate calcaneal or heel ultrasound is done if the patient is immobile.

The DEXA scan is recommended in average risk women at age sixty-five. The National Osteoporotic Foundation recommends screening in men at age seventy. High-risk patients on chronic corticosteroids can start at age fifty. The test is reported using T-scores. Scores greater than -1.5 are normal. Those between -1.5 to -2.5 have osteopenia or brittle bones. Those less than -2.5 are deemed osteoporotic. Fracture risk assessment tool (FRAX) calculators also prognosticate the ten-year probability of a fracture in the hip or other major location. Treatment is also advised for patients whose ten-year risk of a major fracture is equal to or greater than 20 percent, or whose ten-year risk of a hip fracture is greater than 3 percent.

Persons with brittle or osteopenic bones should consume at least 800 IU of Vitamin D and 1200 mg of calcium daily. If osteoporosis is diagnosed, treatment includes bisphosphonates. Bisphosphonates can be given orally in a once-weekly pill or intravenously every year. These medications inhibit the activity of several special bone cleaving cells termed osteoclasts. The medicines can irritate the lining of food pipe, or the esophagus, so should be taken with an eight-ounce glass of water. They must not recline for at least one hour after taking the pill.

Important side effects include atypical fractures of the hip joint and bony jaw destruction called osteonecrosis.

Patients with reduced renal function are often treated twice annually with subcutaneously injected Prolia or Denosumab.

The most feared complication of osteoporosis is a fall. While we have all taken a tumble as a child, shaken it off, and kept on going, this is not always the case after age sixty-five. Falls have such a prominent place in the comprehensive geriatric evaluation of seniors that they should be asked about at every doctor's visit. Some patients disregard and downplay near falls and stumbles and unknowingly forget to inform their doctors. Sassy seniors have had a paradigm shift as it relates to falls. After sitting with their geriatrician and having important conversations, these seniors know the implications of a fall.

At one of my prior clinics, there was a long corridor. I absolutely enjoyed watching my seniors vogue down the runway to my examination room. Many would vivaciously dance for me while my nurses ecstatically cheered them on. Other patients gave their sexiest struts using their cane like a stage prop rather than an intended assistive device! I truly enjoy greeting and spending time with my patients. However, I am doing something more subtle each time they come in to see me.

At Harvard, we were trained to examine gait speed and the stride of the patient's feet. Research has shown that reduced gait speed is correlated with increased mortality. This may seem intuitive because gait results from an intricate interplay between so many organ systems—the muscular, sensory (i.e., vision), nervous, respiratory, and cardiac. A person who walks slower is doing this because their systems are also slowing down. Gait speeds less than 0.6m/s are correlated with increased mortality.

Antalgic or limping gaits may signal arthritic hip pain. Wide-based or ataxic gaits may indicate problems in the cerebellum or damage to the peripheral nerves from diabetes or alcohol dependence. Patients like Muhammad Ali with Parkinson's have deficits in dopamine. They have a classic festinant and shuffling gait.

Fall risks are broadly categorized into those inherent and external factors. I always interrogate my patients about the presence of drop cords, pets, and throw rugs. Vision is integral to movement. A patient that loses depth perception or peripheral field of view from glaucoma or their central visual field from macular degeneration increases their fall risk. A trip to the bathroom late at night can be very menacing. I ensure that we discuss the use of sturdy shower benches, installation of handrails, use of robust bath-tub grip mats, and avoidance of wet tiles. I have discouraged my own parents from ambulating around the home in flip flops. I respectfully caution my patients against precarious behaviors like walking without the use of their designated assistive device or treacherously clinging to furniture edges like a mountain climber who treks up a perilous peak.

As I alluded to earlier, the topic of falls is so expansive because so many organ systems are typically involved. These systems may be iatrogenically affected if seniors are prescribed dangerous cocktails of sedating medications that include combinations of antihistamines, benzodiazepines, and sedating pain medication. They may result from seemingly innocuous medications like diuretics. If a senior takes a water pill but reduces their fluid intake from an illness or from ongoing losses from vomiting, he or she can suffer significant drops in the pressure on sitting to standing. This drop in pressure is termed orthostatic hypotension and can contribute significantly to falling. For this reason, geriatricians who have patients that fall immediately re-create the fall scene like a crime detective to determine if medications and orthostasis are one of the potential suspects!

Sassy and savvy seniors treasure and highly value their independence. They grasp the startling reality that one single fall can result in a fracture, hospitalization, rehabilitation placement, and increased one-year mortality risk. They operate from a preventative mindset. If their Vitamin D levels are well below 30ng/ml they work with their geriatricians to replete the stores. They have educated themselves about the fact that muscle strengthening, and balance are critical in preventing falls. Many are faithful in performing daily stretching exercises such as chair yoga and even Tai Chi.

I cannot stop boasting about the benefits of Tai Chi. This ancient Chinese martial art reprograms the body by having the person in engage in focused repetitive rhythmic movements of the body. The exercises are paired with guided visual imagery. Participants focus on weight shifting and coordination. They utilize meditation and deep breathing while they develop their core muscles and balance. I have personally enrolled many of my patients in this exercise form and witnessed their transformation.

CHAPTER 8

UNLOCKING THE ROYAL CODES: SAVVY SENIORS KNOW THEIR NUMBERS

Where should I aim to keep my blood pressure and blood glucose/sugar as I age? Harvard Professor Lewis Lipsitz also coined the term *post prandial hypotension* to describe the sometimes-drastic drop in blood pressure that occurs after having a large carbohydrate rich meal. The blood vessels in the brain become more rigid with age. This loss of pliability makes it difficult for the vessels to autoregulate and respond to changes in blood flow. Therefore, a drastic reduction in perfusion to the brain will have greater effects in an older person. The American Geriatrics Society and US Preventative Task Force have both relaxed the hypertensive targets in seniors. The goal for blood pressure control is less than 150/90. Other regulatory bodies support the results of the Systolic Blood Pressure Intervention (SPRINT) mind trial, which concluded that achieving a more stringent target of 130/80 or less improves mortality.

I often tell my patients that we can aim to obtain pressures of less than 130/80. This goal should not come at the expense of orthostasis where a patient's systolic blood pressure drops by twenty points or more when moving from sitting to standing. Conversely it is also diagnosed if the patient's diastolic blood pressure decreases by more than 10 points when moving from sitting to standing over a three-minute period. Orthostasis can result in disequilibrium and increased risk of falls.

As the comforts and extremes of Western dieting continue to loom, the prevalence of Type 2 diabetes mellitus in seniors continues to soar. Lack of dietary education, cultural and ethnic differences in diet, coupled with more sedentary lifestyle especially during this new era of COVID can conflate the surge of Type 2 diabetes. Type 2 diabetes mellitus is a state of hyperglycemia that results from the body's resistance to insulin. In contrast to Type 1 diabetics, who fail to produce substantial amounts of insulin in their pancreatic beta cells, persons with Type 2 DM are insensitive to the insulin hormones they produce. This relative insensitivity is insidious. It is the reason why primary care physicians begin diabetic screening in patients over eighteen with a body mass index greater than twenty-five.

Diabetes mellitus is particularly destructive because the constant milieu of glucose eventually wreaks havoc on the micro and macrovascular vessels of the body. Excessive concentrations of glucose can accumulate in the lens of the eyes. This accelerates the formation of cataracts. I often describe having cataracts as trying to see through a cloudy, foggy mirror.

Cataracts reduce the peripheral field of view. Most patients typically find it extremely difficult to drive at night. Reflecting headlights from oncoming vehicles produce a blinding glare. Patients with cataracts often limit their driving to daytime. They also tend to avoid driving in inclement weather conditions such as rain or snow. So important is vision to a patient's sense of independence that many will consent to cataract removal. This surgery is relatively low risk. It is performed in the office under local anesthesia. Patients require an escort once the procedure is completed.

When large amounts of glucose deposit in the vessels, ocular blood vessel walls begin to harden. Blood flow to the retina is reduced. This causes a compensatory increase in the network of vessels that perfuse the retina. The formation of this complex meshwork is termed neovascularization. It can lead to the sensation of black spots or floaters in the patient's field of view. If perfusion to the retina is not improved, the person can eventually lose their vision altogether. This is the most feared complication of diabetic retinopathy.

Savvy seniors are taught from day one about the importance of their annual ophthalmic examination. During their annual examination, cataracts and other diabetic changes in the eyes can be identified. If neovascularization is diagnosed, surgical interventions can be explored. The most common procedure is laser surgery. Here the ophthalmologist applies laser heat to the leaky blood vessels at the posterior of the eye. The heat coagulates the regions of leaking in the vessels. Laser coagulation can be repeated.

Damage to the larger blood vessels such as the coronaries, carotids, and lower extremity arteries can result in myocardial infarctions, carotid stenoses, and peripheral vascular diseases respectfully. Carotid blockages can set the stage for debilitating strokes. I evaluate my patients for carotid stenoses by listening to each carotid artery in their neck while they inhale. Blockages in the carotid lead to reduced blood flow. This creates turbulence and produces an audible murmur called a carotid bruit that can be auscultated during the physical examination.

Prompt recognition of a carotid bruit is integral. Patients can undergo a carotid ultrasound of the neck to determine the percentage of obstruction. Geriatricians adhere to the North American Symptomatic Carotid Endarterectomy Trial (NASCET) criteria to determine which patients can be medically managed versus those who require surgical correction. Vessel blockages that are less than 50 percent are treated by managing the patient's hypertension and cholesterol. Surgery is not performed if a patient already has full 100 percent blockage of the carotid artery. Most patients are placed on a cholesterol medication called a statin and a baby aspirin. This approach also holds true for patients with 50-69 percent vessel blockage. This last category of patients is evaluated systematically with yearly carotid ultrasounds.

Persons whose carotid vessel blockage is between 70-99 percent are evaluated for surgery. The two main options are carotid angioplasty where a stent is inserted to dilate the artery. The more preferred procedure is a carotid endarterectomy or CEA. This procedure is performed by a skilled vascular surgeon.

Sub-optimally controlled diabetes can also place a patient at a greater risk for ulcers of the lower extremities. Many patients with poorly controlled diabetes report excruciating burning pain in their feet. "Doc, it feels like I am walking on tacks or coals of fire!" This condition is termed painful diabetic neuropathy. The high glucose concentrations in the blood also wreak havoc on the nerve endings in the upper and lower extremities. Patients experience the stocking and glove phenomenon when they battle with unremitting pain in the hands and feet. Most patients get some relief by rubbing the affected regions with a pepper containing ointment called Capsaicin. Others require oral medications for nerve pain such as Gabapentin and pregabalin or Lyrica.

Not only does poorly controlled glucose lead to nerve pain, high concentrations of glucose can also impair the sensation in the nerves to travelling to hands and feet. Patients may also develop numbness in the peripheries.

Anesthesia in the feet is significant because patients are unable to appreciate their surroundings. Patients can be blissfully unaware of any injury to their soles. I can remember several unfortunate instances where a patient ended up with a severe infection of the foot from an innocuous heel stick. Diabetes impairs the immune system's ability to fight infections. Poorly healing diabetic ulcers can be a harbinger for eventual toe or foot amputations. For these reasons, geriatricians always meticulously inspect the feet of their diabetic patients. They also ensure that diabetic patients have their yearly preventative visit with the podiatrist.

In the last ten years of practice, I have had the privilege of meeting a wide kaleidoscope of patients. The constant feature of savvy seniors is that they are very judicious and conscientious about their diabetic follow-up. They are well versed in knowing and tracking their hemoglobin A1c values, they understand the significance of both hypo and hyperglycemia. They realize that suboptimal diabetic control can lead to end stage renal disease and dialysis, worsening pain and peripheral neuropathy and feared cerebrovascular accidents and heart attacks.

Diabetic management involves careful tracking of glucose values. When patients wake up, their fasting sugars should be between 80-130mg/dl. Throughout the day, as a person eats, their glucose values will increase. Ideally the desired the glucose reading before each remaining meal should be 140-180mg/dl. Patients and doctors can estimate their average glucose control over a ninety-day period using the hemoglobin A1c. This value converts the pre and post prandial blood glucose into a single or double digit. This is a laboratory test that is ordered by the treating physician.

Diabetes can be diagnosed if a patient has hemoglobin A1c values that are greater than or equal to 6.5 on two separate occasions. Prediabetes is diagnosed if the A1c value falls in the range of 5.7 to 6.4. Patients with prediabetes are educated about the need for lifestyle interventions. These include increased physical activity and attention to observing a lower carbohydrate rich diet plan. Prediabetics may be encouraged to attend diabetes education classes where they can learn important culinary tips.

It may seem intuitive that physicians would want patients to have the lowest A1c value possible. Geriatricians have mastered the art of looking at each patient holistically. I agree I do get excited when my patient's A1c values are less than 7. However, I must temper this excitement if it comes at the cost of them experiencing dangerously low day to day sugars. Patients with labile sugars and repeated episodes of low sugars can be evaluated for a continuous glucose monitoring device.

Hypoglycemia occurs when the glucose is less than 70 mg/ml. It is characterized by marked sweating, dizziness, altered mentation, and even a coma like state.

Hypoglycemia has led to many preventable emergency room visits for seniors. To minimize the occurrence of hypoglycemia, patients and their families are taught how to recognize the symptoms and how to respond. Some respond by administering a carbohydrate rich beverage, ingesting a glucose tablet, or in extreme cases injecting a hormone called glucagon into the patient's muscle. This hormone is made naturally in the pancreas and serves to elevate glucose levels.

So important is the risk of hypoglycemia detection that I always encourage my patients to demonstrate their technique for drawing up insulin. In one unforgettable case, my senior understood our treatment plan. However, due to significant visual impairments, he was drawing up twice the amount of prescribed insulin units. We quickly recognized this and adjusted our treatment strategy with the assistance of his caregiver.

Savvy seniors know that A1c targets vary according to patients. Fit and healthy seniors over sixty-five aim to have an A1c that is less than 7.5. Values lower than 7 are ideal if they do not expose the patient to the risk of hypoglycemia. Seniors with severe chronic comorbidities aim for A1c values under 8 while those nearing end of life with terminal diseases have less stringent targets of less than 9.

CHAPTER 9

NAVIGATING THE HOSPITAL SYSTEM

Savvy seniors select physicians and geriatricians who understand both the necessity of an appropriate hospitalization and the hazards of a preventable one. I am of the utmost belief that hospitalizations are justifiable and necessary when all outpatient measures to stabilize a chronic condition have failed. Let me be clear, a patient should never be diverted away from the hospital in life threatening situations.

An emergency room visit and ensuing hospitalization is expected when a patient presents with an acute event. This can include, for example, a new onset stroke (cerebrovascular accident); heart attack (myocardial infarction), difficulty breathing from an exacerbation of COPD, or rip-roaring blood stream infection termed septicemia.

I always make it a point to instruct patients to go to the emergency room if they develop an acute life-threatening event. Where it is possible, I will coordinate the transfer directly from the office to the emergency room or from home to the hospital. During this transition of care, I personally speak directly to the attending emergency room physician. In this conversation, I provide a succinct but focused summary of my patient. I will outline all the measures and interventions that were taken before transfer. This doctor-to-doctor verbal communication has made the transition of care very smooth for patients and families who are already anxious as their loved one is rushed off and whisked away into an ambulance with blaring sirens and flashing lights.

Patients and their families gain a deep sense of relief when their geriatrician personally makes it a point to coordinate the emergency room transfer. As an internist, I have also followed my patients while in the hospital and obtained updates in their status. Hospitals and emergency rooms can be nerve wracking to seniors and their loved ones.

So why is there no place like home? As much as I enjoy the acuity and instant gratification of seeing my patients rebound and recuperate from an acute event in the hospital, I recognize that hospitals have their own share of risks. The greatest hazards of hospitalization for a geriatrician are the risks of delirium, nosocomial or hospital acquired infection, polypharmacy, and deconditioning.

Research indicates that within two hours of being immobilized on a hospital bed, the muscles of a senior begin to atrophy. Did I just say after two hours? Yes, you read that correctly! Every hour a patient is lying supine and not moving he or she is suffering muscle loss. This is the reason why all geriatricians are relentless in ensuring that hospitalized patients get out of bed and into a chair as soon as possible. It is also the reason why a physical therapy consultation from day one of admission is key. The old adage, "if you don't move it, you will lose it," holds true.

Movement not only helps with lung aeration and bowel motility, but it also prevents the risk of developing decubitus ulcers or blood clots from immobility. Savvy seniors have been educated that every day spent in bed takes two weeks to improve their muscle strength. This severe deconditioning can lead to falls and fractures. Without comprehensive physical therapy, many seniors never regain their premorbid level of functioning by the time they are ready for discharge from the hospital (Creditor, 1933).

The art of geriatric co-management was pioneered by Professor Emeritus Richard Besdine. He holds the distinction of developing the Harvard Geriatric Fellowship. Over his fifty- plus years in the field of Geriatrics he has been an outspoken supporter for seniors. Now at eighty years young, this fierce advocate has no plans of stopping.

During my days as a geriatric fellow at Harvard, I always remembered my orthopedic rotation at The Brigham and Women's Hospital. I especially enjoyed this rotation because I got to collaborate with the orthopedic surgeons as they did the pre-surgical planning for their geriatric patients. After determining that the patient was medically stable to undergo the procedure—often a hip replacement—we would be asked to provide an effective postoperative plan to minimize the risk of delirium.

If you've had a loved one over sixty-five in the hospital, you may have gotten a phone call that he or she may have been acting more confused since hospitalization. Delirium is a geriatric condition that was pioneered and developed nearly four decades ago by guru Dr. Sharon Inouye. About seven million patients annually succumb to this condition. It has led to expenditures of 143 billion dollars. Failure to promptly recognize it can result in prolonged hospitalization and untoward effects. This geriatric syndrome is the bread and butter of geriatrics, so much so that all medical students are taught to diagnose it.

Delirium is a sudden, confusional state with four distinct characteristics. It happens acutely. Patients demonstrate inattention, disorganized thought patterns, and an altered mentation. This hyperactive delirium contrasts to a hypoactive form where the converse is true. The patient may sleep more and interact less. Hypoactive delirium can be easily missed by a well-intentioned medical team if it attributed to ongoing fatigue.

So profound was Dr. Sharon Inouye's trailblazing contribution to our understanding of delirium that many hospitals have implemented mandatory protocols for delirium detection and management. These protocols educate medical staff on identifying risk factors for delirium.

These can be broadly classified into patient specific/intrinsic and environmental or extrinsic factors.

Intrinsic risks are a history of dementia, sub-optimally managed pain, electrolyte disturbances, and baseline sensory deficits just to name a few. The profound effect of sensory deprivation on a patient's orientation is the reason I encourage families to ensure that hospitalized patients have access to their eyeglasses and hearing aids. All too often, an unfamiliar hospital setting can wreak havoc on a senior.

Medications are also an iatrogenic cause of delirium. Certain drug classes like benzodiazepines, anticholinergics, and analgesics can cause confusion. All astute geriatricians immediately perform a careful medication reconciliation when examining a patient who is acutely delirious. We always want to know which medicines were administered in the last twenty-four hours. Once a thorough medication reconciliation is completed, the patient is assessed for any organic causes of confusion.

One common cause is untreated or suboptimally treated pain. Patients who require pain medication should have access to scheduled dosing versus as needed to keep them well above the pain curve. Pain may also result from less innocuous causes. Two often overlooked etiologies are fecal impaction and urinary retention.

I always insist that my medical residents perform a bedside bladder scan to determine if a patient is developing pain from acute urinary retention. If this is the case, placement of foley catheter can bring instant relief and improvement in symptoms. The agitation and confusion that is characteristic of delirium may also result from a simmering infection. In fact, patients who are showing signs of sepsis may demonstrate hypoactive delirium. They may appear more lethargic and engage less with family and nursing staff. It is imperative that patients are screened for potential infections, including urinary tract infections, aspiration pneumonias, or infected decubitus ulcers.

The management of delirium involves immediate recognition of its trigger, and daily prevention. Daily orientation is critical. Nurses, aides, and physicians are reminded to utilize white boards and clocks that can remind patients about the time of day. This is key since many patients tend to sundown or become more confused as the nighttime approaches. With the visitor restrictions that have started with the onset of COVID-19, many patients are unable to see the reassuring faces of their loved ones in person. The medical team must collaborate daily to ensure that the patient is oriented and that sleep wake cycles are maintained. The latter is achieved by minimizing frequent and unnecessary blood draws and vital checks if the patient is resting comfortably.

If these strategies fail and a patient does become delirious, their agitation can pose a risk to their health and safety and others. Conservative measures are often employed with the use of a sitter in the room, attention to scheduled pain medications, etc. Antipsychotics are the last resort for all geriatricians and internists alike. An antipsychotic is a dopamine blocking agent that is used to treat delirium in cases where the patient's behavior poses a threat to their ongoing care. Antipsychotics are divided broadly in two different classes, older formulations called typical antipsychotics and newer formulations called atypical antipsychotics.

Typical antipsychotics include Haldol and Clozapine. Newer atypical drugs include Risperdal and Quetiapine or Seroquel. Typical antipsychotics have more dopamine blockage, while atypical antipsychotics lead to less dopamine receptor blockade in the brain. Typical antipsychotics have a greater risk of neuroleptic malignant syndrome. This is a medical emergency caused by excessive blockage of the dopamine receptor in the brain. These receptors help to coordinate muscle movement. When they become paralyzed, patients develop sustained muscle contractions called dystonia. The symptoms are associated with fevers and confusion. It is treated by administering a drug called Dantrolene.

Delirium treatment is an off-label use of antipsychotics. Patients and families are educated that these drugs do have the potential to increase the risk of a stroke or prolongation the QT interval on the heart's electrocardiogram.

The QT interval is measured in milliseconds and represents the time from the contraction of the heart to its relaxation. The normal QT interval in men is 440ms or less and women is 460ms or less. Longer QT intervals can lead to a potentially fatal cardiac rhythm called Torsades de pointes (twisting of the points), which can eventually result in cardiac arrest.

NAVIGATING YOUR HOSPITAL STAY LIKE A BOSS

While there is no place like home, if you are a sassy senior and you are admitted to the hospital, you can still continue to heal like a boss. First, come to the hospital with an updated medication list. Ensure you or your loved one has important information that is readily accessible for the emergency room doctor. This information includes the date and reason for last hospitalizations, especially if these occurred within the last year. Having scanned copies of imaging like MRIs and CT scans and electronic laboratory results can greatly accelerate the triage process.

Always ensure that your outpatient doctor is immediately notified when you are admitted to the hospital. Savvy seniors go the extra mile by insisting that their attending physicians contact their primary care doctor for pertinent medical history, even while they are in the hospital. This practice is a true boss move and can mean the difference between a lengthier and costlier hospital stay due to duplicate testing by your hospitalist.

Sassy and savvy seniors heal like a boss because they remain intentional. They are not afraid to ask questions to their health care team. They have a trusted confidante who is knowledgeable about their hospitalization and can advocate on their behalf if they are unable to. They minimize the risk of delirium by ensuring they have access to their hearing aids and glasses. They are militant with getting out of bed to a chair and untethering themselves from unnecessary foley catheters and intravenous lines. Early mobility reduces the risk of skin ulcers and overall physical deconditioning. They are actively involved with their care team in discussing the best place for their rehabilitation, be it at a facility or at home. These individuals refuse to let a hospitalization upend their goal of aging like true royalty.

CHAPTER 10

HOW MY SASSY SENIORS TAUGHT ME TO AGE LIKE ROYALTY

If you've made it to this point of the book, let me warn you. It's about to get spicy. One of the reasons that I enjoy working with seniors is because of the rich, diverse variety. Many a time I have sat at their proverbial feet at the conclusion of our appointment and gleaned so much wisdom from their life experiences. My seniors often view me as their fairy granddaughter, with a jacket and stethoscope.

Truth be told, I like it. They always seem to check in on me to ensure that I am doing ok. As I reflect, I become teary-eyed, reminiscing on saved voice messages they would leave on my cell phone wishing me a Merry Christmas. I can recall beautifully hand-decorated birthday banners strewn along the walls to surprise me when I exited a room. I remember one of my dearest gems, Mrs. B., who brought in a massive mouthwatering birthday cake enshrined with a huge replica of my face. To say I was awestruck is an understatement.

In addition to having them recount harrowing stories of civil rights marches and even World War II experiences, the things that I treasure most are the lessons on the secrets of aging like royalty. These are finding purpose in God, self-love, and dying empty.

FINDING PURPOSE IN GOD

At 5:30 A.M., I rise for devotions and timely meditation with God. At 6:30 A.M., when my mind is fresh and renewed, I open my laptop and begin typing. On a good day, I can become inundated with so many ideas that this writing can spill into 7:00 A.M. At that time, I begin to get dressed and ready to arrive for work promptly at 8:00 A.M.

The hurried, frantic, day to day demands of medicine can become challenging. From checking emails to responding to patient and family phone calls, to calling in medications, seeing patients, wrestling with insurance companies, and precepting medical residents, the days often merge into each other. Many of my colleagues often joke that after Monday, the week seems to spin on in a vertiginous blur. Against this backdrop and the reality that you are dealing with life and death, the pursuit of medicine can sometimes take its toll. The best doctors can never please everyone 100 percent of the time.

Patients may never know the times we have foregone milestone anniversaries with families, worked tirelessly through lunch breaks, and coordinated care, even while on vacation, to ensure that they would be getting optimal outcomes. In a time where many physicians are becoming disenchanted with the bureaucracy of medicine, physically and mentally burnt out, and jaded by the once altruistic ideals of medicine, I cling to the truths that my seniors have taught me. Never take for granted the gift of knowledge with which God has endowed you.

The ability to understand the complexities of a human body that is fearfully and wonderfully made by its Omnipotent Creator should never be taken lightly. My patients have taught me the adage that people really do not care how much you know until they know how much you care. As physicians, we must remember the purpose behind this calling. The reason why we fell in love with this specialty. The reason why we sacrificed in some cases—relationships, parties, escapades—throughout various stages of our training. That sacrifice was to become the best physician that we can, so that we can help our patients in their neediest hours.

Behind the closed examination room door is a hallowed sanctuary where patients bare their deepest pains, fears, joys, and frustrations. While my duty primarily is to be their doctor, I have acted as a marriage counselor to couples on the brink of divorce. Beyond the oath of confidentiality that we all take as physicians, I treasure this vulnerability and privilege of witnessing amazing milestone events in their lives.

Patients have shared secrets with me that they will never dream of sharing even with their family members. They bring in pictures and WhatsApp videos of their grandchildren taking their very first steps. I remember encouraging a patient to take a bold leap of faith and change career paths. Together we revamped his resume, did an online job search, and even conducted a mock interview session so he would be ready for the big interview day. Their look of gratitude is just what the doctor ordered!

As a Christian physician I approach my patients holistically. I appreciate the fact that health flows from the balance between the patient's mind and emotions, physical body, and inner spirit. If I treat someone's diabetes without addressing deeper psychosocial issues, I will leave them anchored in despair.

Before the COVID-19 pandemic, many of us were like hamsters on the spinning wheel of life. We were eagerly darting off to the next assignment, giving ourselves little time to pause, reflect, and truly see each other. Like so many, COVID-19 and 2020 allowed me to pause, reset, and refocus. I have developed an even deeper regard and respect for the practice of medicine. I recognize that God has allowed us to practice in the most unprecedented time in modern history.

One of the quotes I treasure dearly comes from the New King James Bible from the Book of Esther. It says, "who knows whether you have come to the kingdom for such a time as this?" So many have been struck with the ravages of COVID-19. Many have not been able to be with their loved ones during their final hours in the Intensive Care Unit. Others have only been able to listen to their family members by phone as their last shallow breaths of life escape their frail bodies. Many families are hurting and in despair after suffering the loss of several relatives at a time. As a Christian physician, I feel more empowered than ever not to lose sight of the reason behind the gift of medicine. It brings me to a quote engraved on a salutatorian plaque I received from my high school on graduation night. "All around are needs to meet, be God's hands, and heart, and feet!"

I have occasions where I instinctively give a warm hug, or join hands in prayer, or begin to have my patients repeat positive affirmations. I know undoubtedly that the wisdom and prompting to do this is not from me, but from the Holy Spirit, whom I go to for guidance and wisdom daily.

Medicine is a gift that if used in its purest form has the power to rejuvenate, reinvigorate and redirect both physician and patient onto their God-given paths. In teaching a new generation of doctors about caring for seniors, I stress the fact that our job is an honor and privilege. Many of my students often hear me say, "If they took the time to come see us, we will show up in that room with a big smile and we will treat them like our parents!"

LOVE OTHERS THE WAY YOU LOVE YOURSELF

I am deeply committed to my craft, so much so that one of my office managers nicknamed me *the beast* because I would attack every task with an undaunting spirit of excellence. One of my front desk colleagues, Shawna, had also coined the moniker *Keyoncé* which was a tribute to my fierce Beyoncé-like work ethic. I was typically the first physician in the clinic and almost always the last one to leave.

Don't get me wrong, I know that being the best in your field demands unwavering commitment to excellence. One of my most memorable patients, however, was careful to remind me of my need to be as intentional in caring for myself as I was for others. "Dr. Rodgers, baby, if you get sick then who's gonna take care of us?" I remember feeling my eyes well up with tears because as much I tried to muster up superwoman strength weaving from one room to the next with my stethoscope draped over my chest, she saw through me. For the first time a patient saw and spoke to me. She recognized that under the white superwoman cape, and shiny metal stethoscope was a young woman who needed to have her own time for self-care and rejuvenation.

Can I be glaringly honest? One of the reasons that I genuinely enjoy caring for seniors over sixty-five is because their sass and brutal honesty is not for the faint of heart. I could potentially retire if I could get a penny for each time I heard the phrase, "Honey, I'm older now so I'm gonna tell it like it is!" Whenever I hear that phrase, I know that I must sit up straight and put on my big girl trousers. My gems are going to serve me a cold glass of honesty with a sweet and tangy side of sage advice.

One of the greatest sources of interest to a small population of my patients is my romantic life. Yes, you read that correctly! Sexy, savvy, sassy seniors want to ensure their doctors are enjoying all facets of life too. My sister would lay in stitches laughing hysterically as I would recount their assessment and management plan for my relationship status.

Some would recommend various dating sites for me while I completed their prescriptions. One patient had offered to arrange a date with her young grandson. This was her version of Tinder, and her grandson was nearly twenty years my junior. Though I never accepted the offer, I was tickled because I knew the gesture was well meaning.

Another patient was determined that she wanted to add some sizzle to my wardrobe, and she truly meant it. I recall the day she strolled in with a pink Victoria's Secret giftbag containing "a little number that would help me get my groove back!" Truthfully, I hadn't realized that in the day-to-day routine of medicine, like Stella, I had somehow lost my groove. I could not believe what I saw as I peered into the bag. She stood and waited calmly for me to look inside. I was speechless. She whispered, "Dr.

Rodgers, I may be older than you, but I can teach you a thing or two, young lady!"

One encounter occurred with a beloved male patient whom I will always remember. I truly enjoyed our visits. At the end of this visit, we had reviewed the goals for his anticoagulation. Today, he respectfully interjected, "Dr. Rodgers, where do you stand in the grocery store?"

I replied, "Well, Mr. P, I'm pretty much in and out of the grocery store." With a coy and mischievous grin, he retorted, "See that's your problem, you have to stand by the meat stand!" After careful introspection, Mr. P had concluded that my lack of romantic escapades was tied to my grocery shopping technique. Perplexed but subtly intrigued I encouraged him to expound. He stated that while he appreciated the great care I provided to my close to four hundred babies, perhaps I would gain even greater joy and satisfaction from offspring of my own. He felt compelled to revamp my haphazard approach to grocery shopping and dating. "The men are at the meat counter, Dr. Rodgers. Please promise me you'll always stand at the meat counter!" Each time I go grocery shopping, I smile as I hear his husky baritone voice when I place my order at the meat counter.

Medicine is demanding. Every other profession too has its demands. At the end of the day, however, we are not our careers. Most times when I am asked to introduce myself, I say that I am Nakeisha. I am an unapologetic

Christian young woman who loves her faith and family. The reactions of some people are priceless when they discover that I am a physician. Truth be told, I can tell a lot about a person if their interaction with me changes drastically only after they discover what I do.

I am especially grateful to my sister, Kathrina, and parents, Hermon and Sylvia, who continue to remind me to enjoy each moment of my life. During COVID, my mother would faithfully call me to ask me if I was relaxing with a hot bath and a good movie. "Girl, put those books and articles down. You cannot sit in front of that computer screen the whole night!" Anyone with a Caribbean mother will know that when they speak, you listen, regardless of your age.

My patients, my family, my friend Genevieve Gomes, and my boss, Dr. Kroker-Bode have all reminded me to create time in my schedule for Nakeisha. This sacred hallow time supplements my early morning prayer and meditation time. I have invested in routine full-body massages with a new masseuse, Ms. T. Another passion I have included in me-time is dance. Years ago, I joined a local YMCA and signed up for belly dancing. The rhythmic well-choreographed workouts enabled us to tone our abdominal muscles while whirling our hips. I'd like to think my Caribbean roots gave me an edge with the latter.

My nurses will tell you that Beyoncé is a fixture on my playlist. Her soundtracks have helped me muster up confidence when I have to deliver bad news to a patient. Her declarations of being a grown woman, a survivor, and even a diva remind me that with God, I can conquer anything. Along with dance, writing has become an important component of me-time. Writing, especially by the beach, is one of the most cathartic experiences.

My parents, primary school teacher, Ms. Moseley, and high school teachers at St. Augustine's College really fostered my passion in literacy. My high school teachers included giants like Mrs. Cooke, Mrs. M. Williams, and Mrs. Thompson. They would cover my essays in a barrage of red pen marks. I am forever grateful for the seeds they planted while I was a teenager.

As God would have it, I met an English Professor named Ms. Carnevale who encouraged me to delve into poetry. In 2000, this led to third prize in a poetry contest, where I met the incomparable global literary icon, the late Dr. Maya Angelou.

Me-time is unique for each and every one of us, but it is so critical. Even Jesus recognized the importance of rest in the Bible. Nakeisha time involves music, dance, poetry. It also involves trips to the spa and days experimenting with a new hairstyle that I saw on Pinterest. My stylist and I enjoy recreating the looks and adding a little unique touch to them. Me-time for you can be whatever you want it to be. For some patients it means reading a good novel, playing with their canine pet, spending time with family, or just soaking in a hot bath. I am thankful to my patients and family for reminding me of the need for me-time. It's a need that I always remind my medical residents about when we sit down quarterly to review their progress.

LIVE EACH DAY LIKE IT'S THE LAST

The Book of Ecclesiastes in the Bible is popular for reminding us that there is a season and time for everything. The Bible further reminds us about the fragility of life. Being a geriatrician is so humbling and yet rewarding because this populace has experienced so much, yet they always seem to acknowledge the sobering fact that tomorrow is not promised to anyone.

Mr. W was a smooth-talking seventy-five-year-old senior who had been transferred to my care. He had a host of medical conditions including atrial fibrillation, congestive heart failure, gout, and debilitating osteoarthritis of the hips. As the months wore on, his mobility worsened. The pain from his arthritis forced him to begin using his cane, which he initially detested, because he was determined to look smooth before his female counterparts. Finally, as the pain worsened, he conceded and began to use his quad cane for greater stability.

As the months wore on, Mr. W's gait speed became slower and the pain in his arthritic hip joint intensified. He became a shell of what he once was. The energetic deep baritone voice that once serenaded us was eventually muffled by pain, which significantly affected the quality of his life. He retreated more and started cancelling appointments because it was becoming too difficult to ambulate.

At this point we had a decision to make about a total hip replacement. He initially declined for fear of his age and the related risks. I was candid to him that his pre-operative risk of mortality was high. However, after an interdisciplinary discussion with his orthopedic surgeon, cardiologist, and myself, we were able to provide Mr. W with all the information he needed to provide informed consent.

"Dr. Rodgers, I'm not scared to die. I've lived a good life. I've travelled the world and met so many wonderful people. I will take the chance on this procedure even if it is my last chance!" I had done pre-operative assessments before. Somehow, this declaration was different. It was a clarion call to me that none of us knows when the end will come. Like Mr. W, it is important to live each day like the last. He survived the surgery. I drove to the hospital to meet him with a big card and huge get-well balloons. When I arrived, I was greeted by that big smile I had come to love, and my serenade as we reminisced more about his days in Motown.

As his nurse entered the room to administer his scheduled dose of pain medications, I remember seeing him beam with pride as he introduced me. "I'd like you to meet my doctor. This is Dr. Rodgers." What was intended to be a short visit turned into two amazing hours. I commended him for his bravery in undergoing the surgery. We reviewed the plan for rehabilitation. The geriatrician and schoolteacher in me reminded him to prevent any postoperative complications.

I reminded him to have his foley catheter removed as soon as possible to prevent a urinary tract infection. I encouraged him to use his bedside incentive spirometer several times a day. This would strengthen his diaphragm, increase his lung expansion, and reduce the risk of postoperative pneumonia and regions of lung deflation called atelectasis. We ensured that his pain medication was supplemented with a laxative to reduce the risk of opioid-induced constipation. Most importantly, I reminded him of the hazards of hospitalization. The biggest hazard was deconditioning. He was encouraged to participate in the hospital physical therapy exercises and to move from bed to chair as much as possible to strengthen his body.

As I enter different stages of life, saying goodbye to my patients is always one of the hardest things I have to do. It involves many nights of tears and what ifs. I had grown accustomed to managing their medical needs. One of the biggest lessons they reminded me of, however, is that because life is not promised, we must feed our faith and starve our fears. Living a life of God-filled purpose involves meeting new challenges. Like Mr. W, we will not always be 100 percent certain of the outcome, but we must launch into the deep.

CONCLUSION

This book is my launch. As a physician, I get to care for people from so many walks of life. One of the things that I have seen is that so many people medically perish and fail to live their best lives from simple lack of knowledge. True, we live in a modern day technologically savvy age where the answer to any question is literally under our fingertips on a keyboard search. However, due to disparities in access and the lack of time to fully teach, many patients lack the education they need to become advocates for themselves and for their families. *Age Like Royalty* was my God-given mandate and response to seniors to provide them with the information they need to lead rich, independent lives.

If you are reading this book, this is a clarion call to you as well. If there is a dream in your heart that God has placed, take the first step by recognizing it. Like the New King James Bible book Habakkuk states, "Write the vision and make it plain." Ask God for guidance and be receptive when He responds. His Divine providence often comes in the form of people, mentors, books, and opportunities.

Like the late great Dr. Myles Munroe, once you discover God's distinct purpose for you, your duty is to step out and become so phenomenal that your service to humanity is undeniable. Then you will be able to truly reign and age like royalty!

AFTERWORD

I am so appreciative of the coaching I received from Dr. Draion Burch, who helped me to explore the gift of writing God has placed inside of me. This book is a tribute to the patients who literally gave their lives to empower me with the secrets behind successful aging. The road to aging is one that I too will travel someday. I am grateful to have the royal roadmap to direct me at every step.

REFERENCES

Altman, D., and W. Frist. 2015. "Medicare and Medicaid at 50 years Perspectives of Beneficiaries, Health care professionals and institutions, and policy Makers." *Journal of American Medical Association,* 314, no. 4 (July 28, 2015).

Creditor, Mortan Dr. 1993. Annals of Internal Medicine. 11 no. 3. (February 1993).

Durso, Samuel et al. 2013. *Geriatrics Review Syllabus,* 8th ed. New York: American Geriatrics Society Publishing, 2013.

Jenkins, JoAnn. 2016. *Disrupt Aging.* New York: Public Affairs, 2016.

Ouslander, J. et al. 2018. *Essentials of Clinical Geriatrics,* 8th ed. McGraw Hill Education, 2018.

Semmens, Shana. 2019. "CPR Advice for helping patients and families decide." *Elder Care, University of Arizona Center on Aging.* August 2019. https://www.uofazcenteronaging.com/care-sheet/providers/cpr-advice-helping-patients-and-families-decide.

ABOUT THE AUTHOR

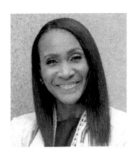

Dr. Nakeisha Raquel Rodgers is an internist and geriatrician who hails from Nassau, Bahamas. The youngest of six, she credits her parents, Hermon and Sylvia Rodgers, for helping her hone her God-given gift of teaching. After earning degrees from the University of the Bahamas, Acadia University, and the University of the West Indies, she completed her residency at Yale New Haven Bridgeport Hospital and her geriatric training at Harvard Medical School.

Dr. Nakeisha currently serves as assistant clinical professor of internal medicine and geriatrics and is the assistant director of the FSU Internal Medicine Residency Clinic in Tallahassee, Florida. There, she earned the prestigious 2020 Faculty of the Year Award.

A devout Christian, her faith and belief in Jesus Christ are central to who she is. Dr. Nakeisha teaches Sunday school in the Bahamas and enjoys the creative arts.